COVID-19 Through the Lens of Mental Health in India

This book provides an in-depth understanding of the impact of COVID-19 on the psychological health of people and communities in India.

Focusing on the current discourse on Mental Health literacy in India, the book also analyses COVID-19-specific health beliefs and their convergences and divergences with COVID-19 protocols and advisories. It discusses the impact of the pandemic on survivors of COVID-19 including their quality of life, psychological well-being, and coping mechanisms while tackling loneliness, loss, and grief. It explores the psychological and social challenges which children have faced during the pandemic and offers techniques to address and adequately manage Mental Health challenges.

Grounded in theoretical and empirical research, this book will be of interest to students, teachers, and researchers of psychology, social psychology, Mental Health and wellness studies, and sociology. It will also be useful for academicians, social workers, healthcare workers, and psychologists.

Tilottama Mukherjee is Associate Professor and Head of the Department of Psychology at the University of Calcutta, India, and a RCI-registered Clinical Psychologist. She has published extensively and has presented her research in national and international conferences on Mental Health and wellness, applied psychology, behaviour therapy, and social psychology.

COVID-19 Through the Lens of Mental Health in India

Present Status and Future Directions

Edited by
Tilottama Mukherjee

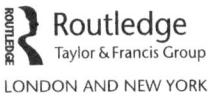
Routledge
Taylor & Francis Group

LONDON AND NEW YORK

First published 2023
by Routledge
4 Park Square, Milton Park, Abingdon, Oxon OX14 4RN

and by Routledge
605 Third Avenue, New York, NY 10158

Routledge is an imprint of the Taylor & Francis Group, an informa business

British Library Cataloguing-in-Publication Data
A catalogue record for this book is available from the British Library

ISBN: 978-1-032-22561-6 (hbk)
ISBN: 978-1-032-39109-0 (pbk)
ISBN: 978-1-003-34842-9 (ebk)

DOI: 10.4324/9781003348429

Typeset in Times New Roman
by Apex CoVantage, LLC

Contents

Figures

Tables

Contributors

Urmimala Ghose is a doctoral student at the Humboldt University Berlin, under the doctoral programme conducted by the International Max Planck Research School on the Life Course, Berlin. She is also clinical psychologist, registered with the Rehabilitation Council of India. Her areas of interest are positive psychology, and self in the context of human life course and changing sociohistorical milieu. Other than psychology, she is deeply passionate about Indian music and photography.

Dr. Aniruddha Deb is a practising psychiatrist in the private sector in Kolkata. He has been working as an independent practitioner for more than 25 years. His special area of interest is child and adolescent Mental Health, specifically issues arising out of trauma, chronic stressors such as academic and school pressure which have been mounting over the decades in his work field. He has worked with parents and pedagogues to reduce pressure on children adolescents, particularly on adolescents, because of the abnormal stress they have to go through because of ill-understood changes in that stage of life. He has spoken in national and regional seminars on various Mental Health issues on many occasions.

Dr. Jaseem Koorankot has been a Licensed Clinical Psychologist & Psychotherapist with Solution Focused orientation since 2010. He writes and presents on solution-focused brief therapy, psychotherapy process research, affective neuroscience, career psychology, and psychometric test construction. Dr. Jaseem is currently employed as Assistant Professor & Head at Department of Clinical Psychology, Institute of Mental Health and Neurosciences (IMHANS), Govt. Medical College, Calicut, Kerala, India.

Ms. Avisikta Basu is an Assistant Professor of Applied Psychology, currently working at the Centre for Human Ecology, School of Human Ecology, Tata Institute of Social Sciences, Mumbai. She has completed

M.Phil in Clinical Psychology from the University of Calcutta and also practices as a Clinical Psychologist. Her interest lies in the area of epidemiological aspects of Mental Health. She is also keen on working and exploring the association of performing arts and its association with different aspects of Clinical psychology.

Ms. Turfa Ahmed completed an undergraduate degree in Psychology at Loreto College (Kolkata), and subsequently pursued a Master's degree in Psychology, with specialization in Clinical Psychology from University of Calcutta (Kolkata). She is presently a 2nd year trainee Clinical Psychologist, enrolled in an M.Phil. programme at the University of Calcutta, Kolkata. Her clinical interest areas have included work with children, adolescent and adults with a wide range of Mental Health problems. She primarily uses cognitive behavioural therapy and third wave interventions like Mindfulness in practice. Her research interests involve youth Mental Health and well-being, and third wave behavioural interventions.

Ms. Sukanya Chowdhury is a M.Phil Scholar of Clinical Psychology at the University of Calcutta. Having completed her graduation from Loreto College, she pursued her Masters in Psychology from Calcutta University. Her areas of interest lie in personality disorders, autism spectrum disorder, neuropsychological functioning, social cognition and third wave behavioral intervention. As a clinician and researcher, she works with children and young adults on a daily basis, trying to focus on and bring to light the various factors that affect their Mental Health and help them resolve it. A firm believer of equal rights for all and a Mental Health advocate, Ms. Chowdhury dreams of creating a world where Mental Healthcare is accessible to every citizen and where we speak about mental illness without an ounce of shame and taboo.

Ashmita Mukherjee Manipal Institute of Technology, Udupi, Karnataka: BTech in Electrical and Electronics Engineering final year.

Preface

Two years back, the world was stopped overnight by a minuscule virus wreaking havoc in people's lives. An eternal sense of hopelessness crept into our minds. No one seemed to have a definite idea about the nature of the virus, the lasting effects on our bodies, or how long it would take to disappear from our lives. Anything unknown scares anyone. Living in a constant state of fear and despair was bound to take a toll on our Mental Health. As health professionals around the world cautioned us about the long-lasting physical impact of this disease, a silent, more severe pandemic was brewing among humankind. It was the damaging impact of this global phenomenon on the Mental Health of individuals worldwide. A pandemic of this nature followed by subsequent lockdowns has hardly been witnessed in the last few decades. Thus, it would be fair to assume that it would lead to various Mental Health issues and several other difficulties.

The idea behind this book was to look into the nature of these difficulties and map the landscape of Mental Health problems faced by adults and children in a post-pandemic world. The book comprises empirical studies and review chapters on Mental Health during and after the COVID-19 pandemic hit India. The empirical research covered in this book spans diverse areas of Mental Health.

Chapter 1 addresses the stigma and discrimination people face with Mental Health problems. It discusses relevant findings from an empirical study on the Mental Health stigma and the tendencies of professional help-seeking in the middle of the COVID-19 pandemic. Thus, the stigma around Mental Health has been broadly explored among young, late, and early middle-aged adults. Their subsequent tendency to seek help from Mental Health professionals during the pandemic was also a theme surveyed across the groups of individuals. Such a study adds to the ongoing dialogue around Mental Health literacy in India.

Chapter 2 sheds light on the different COVID-19-specific health beliefs held by Indian adults, viz., perceived susceptibility and severity of the disease, perceived benefits and barriers of performing health behaviours, and self-efficacy of the individuals themselves, as well as the extent to which they comply to the COVID-19 behaviour protocols, especially in the context of the second wave of the pandemic in India. The role of health beliefs and behaviours during the pandemic furthers the discussion on community Mental Health.

Chapter 3 brings forth findings that discuss the impact of COVID-19 on the general health, quality of life, and resilience of COVID-19 survivors from India. An attempt was made to initiate a conversation around the differences in indices of Mental Health between Indian adults who have suffered from COVID-19 and those who did not. The impact of the pandemic was objectively measured among such individuals for that purpose.

Chapter 4 comprises empirical studies that seek to understand how psychosocial factors such as loneliness and cognitive emotion regulation contribute to students' psychological well-being during the pandemic and identify strategies to promote students' well-being during and beyond the pandemic. The cost of bearing with the pandemic has been expensive for the students, indicating poor well-being outcomes. Students have never felt lonelier due to social distance, disruption of academic life, and emotional disturbances. A prevalent issue yet not widely spoken, student Mental Health during the pandemic has also been a theme covered by this book.

Along with focusing on adults and their Mental Health amidst these trying times, *Chapter 5* discusses the difficulties faced by children during the lockdown. The pandemic and subsequent lockdowns have been difficult for all children, especially those with pre-existing mental illnesses. The problems faced by the children and the management strategies that can be implemented in such cases have been talked about at length. Children with neurodevelopmental disorders and other Mental Health problems also add to the burden of care on the primary caregivers. Such children are susceptible to abuse and neglect from families. This chapter urges the stakeholders to address the matter, keeping the context of pandemics in mind.

During the pandemic, psychologists and therapists have had to deal with a new and unique set of challenges raised by the toll of the pandemic on global Mental Health. *Chapter 6* delineates a solution-focused, strength-based approach as a workable model that can empower clients in such times of crisis. The chapter, therefore, adds to the literature on solution-focused practice in India, which is still in the nascent stages. The approach of solution-focused strategies during the pandemic has helped alleviate the Mental Health distress of several individuals, and this chapter presents a workable model for furthering such practices in India.

The book explores the Mental Health scenario in a post-pandemic world. It encourages discussions about a silent but more devastating pandemic that has affected millions of people in India and several other countries.

1 Health Beliefs and Compliance to Health Behaviours During the COVID-19 Pandemic

A Survey Among Indian Adults

Ashmita Mukherjee, Urmimala Ghose and Tilottama Mukherjee

Introduction

Since the end of 2019, the COVID-19 pandemic has made the world witness a major global health crisis yet again. Although China had been its first victim, COVID-19 cases spread to other parts of the world like a wildfire owing to the easy international mobility prevalent in the twenty-first century. Consequently, nations across the globe implemented non-pharmaceutical control measures to avoid the transmission of this disease. These may be at individual level, such as, the use of facemasks, washing, and sanitizing hands at regular intervals, as well as at community level, such as physical distancing. Moreover, governments and health authorities have been disseminating information about the preventive practices through all possible means (Sjödin et al., 2020; Wilder-Smith & Freedman, 2020). India has not been an exception regarding this issue. The Ministry of Health, Government of India, has also implemented strict preventive measures in order to contain the spread of the virus since March 2020, consistent with those prescribed by the World Health Organization. Public awareness programmes about COVID-19 and the means of necessary protection against it are also being conducted through mass media and social media. However, the stringent "lockdown" that had been imposed by the Indian government in March 2020 was withdrawn gradually since June 2020, and the year 2021 is marked by the return of the Indian citizens to their "new normal" life, although with considerable restrictions.

Even though vaccination campaigns have been started in most countries, there is still a long way until every citizen gets access to it especially in developing countries like India. India began its vaccination drives on 16 January 2021, and as of 21 November, 55% of the population has been administered with at least one dose and 29.1% of the population has

DOI: 10.4324/9781003348429-1

been fully vaccinated (Ministry of Health, 2021). Furthermore, researchers have found that the efficacy of vaccination in the prevention of the disease is variable, depending on the type of vaccine used. Recent findings reveal that even vaccinated individuals can still be infected and can spread the virus. Therefore, it is needless to say that community preventive measures have not lost their relevance in effectively controlling the pandemic.

Previous research has identified several factors that can interfere with the enactment of prevention (Friedman & Kern, 2014), and many of them undoubtedly are applicable in the context of the current pandemic. Evidence from previous pandemics show that poor health literacy is related to negative emotions among individuals, which, in turn, can complicate the preventive attempts even more (Person et al., 2004). Individuals are likely to differ on the psychological and behavioural responses that contribute to the prevention and control of the current as well as future health crises. It is necessary to consider every individual to be the most crucial factor in promoting health; and the adaptive or maladaptive behaviours are, to a large extent, determined by one's beliefs, values, tendencies, and habits (Chan et al., 2020). Therefore, understanding the determinants responsible for people's resistance to protective measures against the virus spread is of great importance for the effectiveness of social isolation-based public policies, avoiding or reducing non-adherence to the proposed social controls.

A plethora of models and theories have been proposed by psychologists, sociologists, and anthropologists to explain the different factors of health behaviours, the Health Behaviour Model or HBM (Rosenstock, 1974) being one of the most widely cited among them. It attempts to explain patients' behaviour in the face of an illness or the risk of falling ill (Grosser, 1982). The model provides a general conceptual framework and theoretical guideline for behaviours that have been identified as promoters of health. It consists of a number of relevant constructs as follows: perceived susceptibility, perceived severity, perceived benefits, perceived barriers, self-efficacy, and additionally cues to action (Rosenstock, 1974; Rosenstock et al., 1988). We have used this model as a theoretical framework for our current study, including the first five constructs.

According to the HBM, positive factors increase pro-health behaviours, while negative factors decrease or inhibit them. It posits that people should consider the health threat (e.g. COVID-19) as serious problem so that they should participate in preventive behaviours. It means that they should think themselves to be vulnerable to the threat (perceived susceptibility) and perceive its risks and complications (perceived severity). Moreover, perceiving the effectiveness of preventive behaviour and trying to diminish barriers to preventive behaviour can enhance the possibility of showing these behaviours. Self-efficacy refers to the belief that one can successfully perform a behaviour that will then lead to a desirable outcome. Further, the HBM suggests that a cue or trigger (e.g. symptoms, strategies, or information sources) that supports the implementation of a behaviour is needed for motivating participation in healthy behaviours (Rosenstock, 1974; Rosenstock et al., 1988).

The reason behind the general acceptance and popularity of the health belief model is its high predictive power (Rosenstock et al., 1988). The HBM was first developed in the United State Public Health Service in the 1950s as a possible explanation for participation in medical prevention and disease detection programs (Glanz et al., 2008). Among other uses, this model has been successfully applied to assess diabetes severity (Hurley, 1990), analyse protective factors for bulimia (Grodner, 1991), find determinants for oral health care (Wilson et al., 2018), and study the perception of different cultures on dementias (Sayegh & Knight, 2013). It has also been applied to the MERS-CoV COVID-19 virus infection (Alsulaiman & Rentner, 2018) to understand the compliance with measures recommended by the Saudi Arabian government, a situation resembling the current pandemic. Further, quite a few recent studies have examined the constructs of the HBM in context of the COVID-19 pandemic worldwide. Along with Western countries like Poland (Nowak et al., 2020), studies have been conducted in countries of other parts of the world like Iran (Mirzaei et al., 2021; Shahnazi et al., 2020), Saudi Arabia (Syed et al., 2021), Ethiopia (Yehualashet et al., 2021), and Brazil (Costa, 2020), among others. To our knowledge, only one study has so far been conducted in India (Jose et al., 2021) in this context. However, this study was based on respondents from only one state, that is Kerala. India being a multicultural nation, and different geographical regions being affected by the pandemic at different points of time with different levels of severity, more studies are required to examine the applicability of the HBM to the Indian population with respect to this disease, involving participants across the nation.

In the current chapter, we have detailed the course and results of our research to evaluate the five constructs of HBM as well as the degree of compliance to preventive measures to contain the spread of COVID-19 among the Indian citizens. Additionally, we also examined the degree of association of the HBM constructs with the compliance. Finally, we investigated whether these constructs differed across various sociodemographic groups.

Methods

Participants

Two hundred and seventy one Indian citizens, aged above 18 years, voluntarily participated in the study. Among the participants, about 59.63% (161) were females. Seventy per cent (189) were aged below 30 years. About 51.85% (140) had been staying in West Bengal at the time of conducting the study. The detailed sociodemographic description of the sample is given in Table 1.1.

Materials

Our study employed an information schedule, the COVID-19 Health Beliefs Model Scale (Nowak et al., 2020, adapted from Champion, 1984) and the Compliance with COVID-19 Recommended Behaviours Scale (Kamran et al., 2020).

The information schedule requested certain sociodemographic and COVID-19-specific details from the respondents. To measure health

Table 1.1 Sociodemographic description of the sample (N = 271)

		N	%
Sex	Male	110	40.59
	Female	161	59.41
Age Group	Below 30	189	69.74
	Above 30	82	30.26
Place of Residence	Semi-urban	39	14.39
	Urban	232	85.61
Current State/UT	Other	131	48.34
	West Bengal	140	51.66
Education	Up to graduate	134	49.45
	Postgraduate	137	50.55
Marital Status	Married	73	26.94
	Unmarried	191	70.48
H/O Chronic Illness	Absent	213	78.60
	Present	58	21.40
H/O Contracting COVID-19	Absent	202	74.54
	Present	69	25.46
H/O Death of Any Acquaintance due to COVID-19	Absent	75	27.68
	Present	196	72.32

Source: Author/s

beliefs about the COVID-19 virus (Wave 2), we used the Health Beliefs Model Scale (Nowak et al., 2020, adapted from Champion, 1984). Nowak and colleagues modified (20 items only) the Health Belief Model Scale (Champion, 1984) by substituting the name of the virus (e.g. "The chance that I will get the COVID-19 virus during my lifetime is very high") with other health conditions (e.g. "The chance that I will get the breast cancer during my lifetime is very high") and created 20-item COVID-19 Health Beliefs Scale. The scale captures individual differences in perceived barriers, perceived susceptibility, perceived severity, perceived benefits, and self-efficacy (four items each). Participants indicated how true they believed each item was (1 = definitely not, 4 = definitely yes). The five indices of health beliefs were obtained by averaging the responses to the items of each subscale. The reliability coefficients ranged from 0.60 to 076.

The behaviour compliance was assessed by using the Compliance with COVID-19 Recommended Behaviours Scale (Kamran et al., 2020). It consists of nine statements each of which the respondents have to rate on a seven-point scale, where, 1 equals "Least Observance" and 7 equals "Most Observance." The reliability coefficient for the scale was 0.85.

Data Collection and Study Set-Up

All data were collected through online survey (Google forms), circulated through social media platforms and messaging applications. Participants responded to the questionnaires after giving informed consent. It took approximately 10 to 12 minutes to complete the survey. The data were collected from 1st to 15th June, 2021, towards the end of the second wave of pandemic in India.

Statistical Analyses

Means and standard deviations were computed for each of the variables. The assumptions of normality for the distributions of each of the variables were checked using the Shapiro–Wilk test, revealing the distributions to be done non-normally. Hence, non-parametric tests were conducted for further statistical analyses. Spearman's rho correlation coefficient was determined for each of the HBM constructs with compliance to preventive behaviours. Mann–Whitney U tests were conducted to determine if the various sociodemographic groups differed with respect to the variables under study.

Results

Perceived Susceptibility

The results have demonstrated a relatively lower level of perceived susceptibility (mean ± SD, range: 2.43 ± 0.75, 1–5) about novel COVID-19 virus pandemic in the respondents (Table 1.2). Only 12.9% (probably yes/definitely yes) of respondents had perceived susceptibility of contracting novel COVID-19 virus anytime soon. More than one third (36.5%) of respondents had perception that the chances of getting COVID-19 during their lifetime were very high. Only 19.2% of respondents were of the opinion that compared to the average people, the chance that they would get a COVID-19 virus was extremely high. As low as 7% of the respondents reported of thinking that they were already sick with COVID-19 virus (Table 1.3).

Table 1.2 Descriptive statistics of all the variables measured (N = 271)

Variables Measured	Range of Possible Scores	Mean	Std. Deviation
Perceived Susceptibility	1–5	2.4262	.75437
Perceived Severity	1–5	2.5028	.86696
Perceived Benefits	1–5	3.3072	.93564
Perceived Self-Efficacy	1–5	3.6301	1.00757
Perceived Barriers	1–5	2.0101	.67539
Compliance to Health Behaviours	9–63	47.2472	11.69274

Source: Author/s

Table 1.3 Percentage of respondents endorsing the rating points on each item of the COVID-19 Health Beliefs Model Scale (N = 271)

Domain	Items	Percentage (%) of Respondents Endorsing the Rating Points				
		1	*2*	*3*	*4*	*5*
Perceived Susceptibility	1. I will probably get COVID-19 virus anytime soon.	11.1	37.6	38.4	11.8	1.1
	6. The chance that I will get a COVID-19 virus during my lifetime is very high.	11.4	26.2	25.8	24	12.5
	11. Compared to the average poll, the chance that I will get a COVID-19 virus is extremely high.	17.3	33.9	29.5	14.8	4.4
	16. I think I am already sick with COVID-19 virus.	64.6	19.9	8.5	3.7	3.3

Domain	Items	Percentage (%) of Respondents Endorsing the Rating Points				
		1	*2*	*3*	*4*	*5*
Perceived Severity	2. The mere thought that I may be sick with the COVID-19 virus scares me.	25.5	32.8	5.5	24.7	11.4
	7. If I get COVID-19 virus, I will suffer from various ailments for a long time.	16.2	33.6	30.3	17	3
	12. If I get COVID-19 virus, my whole life will change.	31.7	39.1	18.1	8.1	3
	17. Getting COVID-19 virus is a more serious threat to your health than getting other similar diseases.	19.2	31	19.6	22.1	8.1
Perceived Benefits	3. Frequent washing of my hands allows me not to worry so much about the possibility of infection.	25.5	32.8	5.5	24.7	11.4
	8. Compliance with the recommendations of medical organizations calms me down.	5.9	18.1	14	40.2	21.8
	13. Regularly checking for COVID-19 virus symptoms gives me the confidence that I'm healthy.	18.8	22.9	14	32.1	12.2
	18. My efforts allow me to look calmly into the future, even in a situation in which I develop a COVID-19 virus.	7.4	14	19.2	38.4	21
Perceived Self-Efficacy	4. Reducing contact with other people will reduce the risk of my illness.	6.6	15.1	10	32.8	35.4
	9. Frequent washing of my hands will reduce the risk of my illness.	7.4	16.2	11.4	40.2	24.7
	14. Checking for COVID-19 virus symptoms will allow me to detect it early enough.	10.3	14.8	12.5	40.2	22.1
	19. Even if I will get a COVID-19 virus, thanks to my efforts I will recover.	5.2	12.2	18.5	36.9	27.3

(Continued)

Table 1.3 (Continued)

Domain	Items	Percentage (%) of Respondents Endorsing the Rating Points				
		1	*2*	*3*	*4*	*5*
Barriers	5. I do not have time to apply preventive measures.	68.3	22.9	3	3.3	2.6
	10. I have a hard time remembering to use various methods to prevent COVID-19 virus infection.	44.3	30.6	12.9	10	2.2
	15. My friends and family would laugh at me if I showed that I was concerned about COVID-19 virus.	60.1	24.4	7.4	5.5	2.6
	20. I have more important problems on my mind than dealing with COVID-19 virus.	14.8	25.5	25.1	20.7	14

Source: Author/s

Table 1.4 Percentage of respondents endorsing the rating points on each item of the COVID-19 Recommended Behaviours Scale (N = 271)

Items	Percentage (%) of Respondents Endorsing the Rating Points						
	1	*2*	*3*	*4*	*5*	*6*	*7*
1. Wearing gloves out of home	42	18.6	11.7	10.2	8.3	4.2	4.9
2. Wearing mask out of home	4.5	3.8	3.8	2.3	2.7	7.2	75.8
3. Wearing mask in contact with patients	4.2	4.2	4.5	1.1	1.9	3	81.1
4. Stay at home	4.9	4.2	11		7.6	17.8	22.3	32.2
5. Absence from family and religious ceremonies	4.5	6.1	8		9.1	12.1	20.8	39.4
6. Minimizing presence in the community, such as reducing purchases and administrative and banking visits	4.2	4.9	6.8	9.8	20.1	22.3	31.8
7. Frequent hand washing with soap and water	4.5	5.7	9.1	6.4	11	23.5	39.8
8. Frequent hand washing with soap and water	3	4.2	6.1	8.3	11	21.2	46.2
9. Disinfection of personal items such as keychains, mobile phones, and cars	6.1	8	7.2	8.3	14.4	20.1	36

Source: Author/s

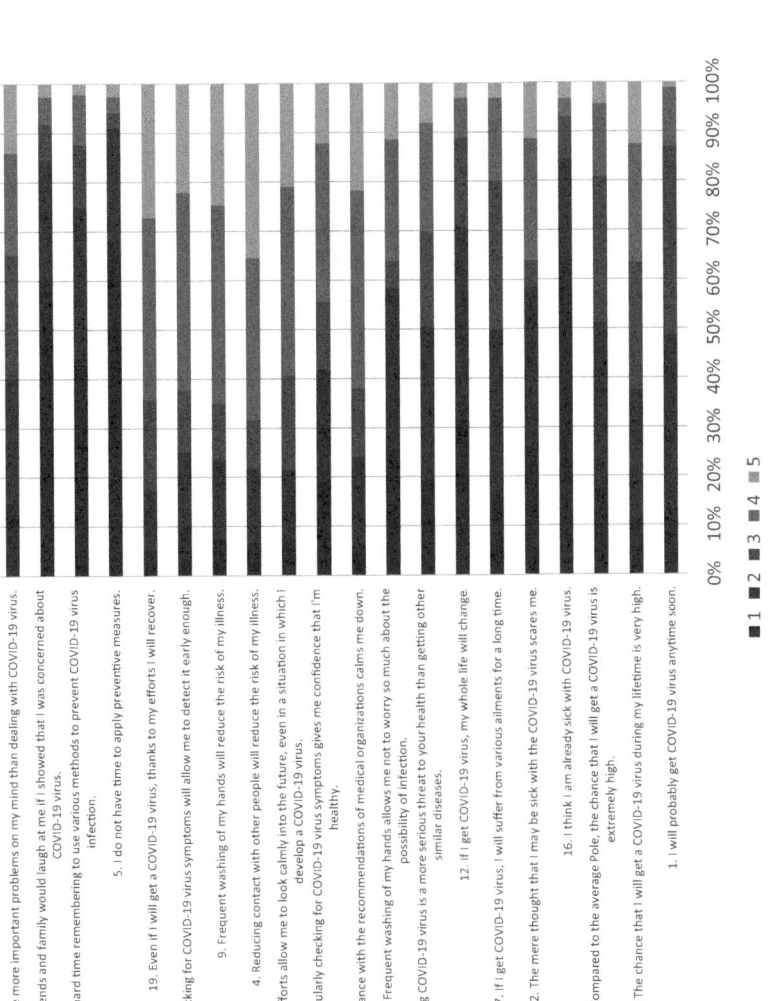

Figure 1.1 Graphical Representation of Percentage of Respondents Endorsing the Rating Points on Each Item of the COVID-19 Health Beliefs Model Scale (N = 271)

Source: Author/s

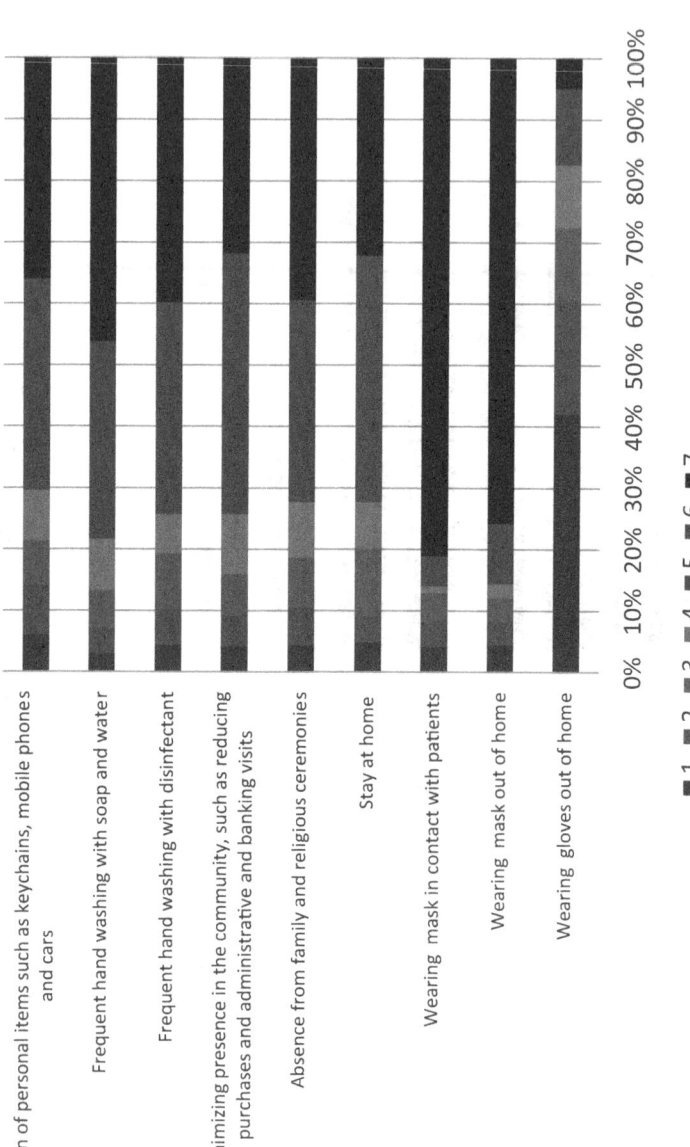

Figure 1.2 Graphical Representation of Percentage of Respondents Endorsing the Rating Points on Each Item of the COVID-19 Recommended Behaviours Scale (N=271)

Source: Author/s

Perceived Severity

The results of perceived severity were also observed at a relatively lower level (mean ± SD, range: 2.50 ± 0.87, 1–5) (Table 1.2). The mere thought that they may be sick with the COVID-19 virus scares 36.1% of the respondents, and 30.2% consider that getting COVID-19 virus is a more serious threat to their health than getting other similar infections. Very low percentages (20% and 11.1%) of respondents think that if they get COVID-19 virus, they will suffer from various ailments for a long time, and they will suffer from various ailments for a long time, respectively (Table 1.3 and Figure 1.1).

Benefits

Perceived benefits were found to be at a relatively higher level (mean ± SD, range: 3.31 ± 0.94, 1–5) (Table 1.2). Majority of the respondents (62%) reported that complying with the preventive measures helps to calm them down. A large proportion (59.4%) perceived that these efforts of compliance allow them to look into the future in a much level-headed manner, even considering the risk of contracting the disease. More than the half of the participants (54.2%) reported that frequent hand-washing habits allow them not to worry so much about the chances of getting COVID-19. About 44.3% believed that self-monitoring the symptoms of COVID regularly helps to make them feel confident about their health condition (Table 1.3 and Figure 1.1).

Perceived Barriers

The results have demonstrated a relatively lower level of perceived barriers (mean ± SD, range: 2.01 ± 0.68, 1–5) about the novel COVID-19 virus pandemic in the respondents (Table 1.2). As low as 5.9% of the respondents reported that they did not have the time to apply preventive measures. Only 8.1% believed that they would be laughed at by their friends and family if they showed their concern about the disease. About 12.9% found it hard to remember complying to the preventive measures. However, a relatively large proportion of the participants (34.7%) reported that they had more important problems on their mind than dealing with COVID-19 (Table 1.3 and Figure 1.1).

Perceived Self-Efficacy

Perceived self-efficacy of the respondents was also observed at a relatively higher level (mean ± SD, range: 3.63 ± 1.01, 1–5) (Table 1.2). Majority of the participants (68.4% and 64.9%) believed that reducing contact with others and frequent hand-washing habits would lower the risk of contracting COVID-19. A large percentage (64.2%) were of the opinion that even in the case of getting the disease, they will recover owing to their efforts in observing proper COVID-19 measures. Respondents (62.3%) also believed that self-monitoring for COVID-19 symptoms would help them detect the disease at an earlier stage (Table 1.3 and Figure 1.1).

Compliance

The results have shown a high level of compliance among respondents in practicing community-protective measures to prevent the spread of COVID-19 virus (mean ± SD, range: 47.53 ± 11.69, 9–63) (Table 1.2). Majority of respondents (agreed/strongly agreed) showed compliance with wearing masks when in contact with parents (86%) as well as wearing mask outside home (85.7%). Most of them also reported of washing their hands frequently with soap and water (78.4%) and with disinfectant (74.3%), staying at home (72.3%), refraining from being physically present in the community (74.2%), and regularly disinfecting personal belongings (70.5%). However, gloves were worn out of home for protection against the virus by a relatively small proportion of the participants (17.4%) (Table 1.4 and Figure 1.2).

Association of Compliance With the HBM Constructs

Modest, yet significant, positive correlation was found between perceived severity and compliance only (Table 1.5). None of the other HBM constructs showed significant associations with compliance of the respondents.

Table 1.5 Spearman's rho correlation coefficients between different components of Health Belief Model (HBM) and compliance to health behaviours (N = 271)

HBM Components	Spearman's Rho
Perceived Susceptibility	0.015
Perceived Severity	0.135*
Perceived Benefits	0.038
Perceived Self-Efficacy	0.104
Perceived Barriers	−0.06

* $p < 0.05$

Source: Author/s

Comparison Across Sociodemographic Groups

The results of comparison of the HBM constructs and compliance are presented in Table 1.6. In the current study, significant differences were observed on the following domains: perceived susceptibility with respect to the current state/UT and history of chronic illness; perceived severity with respect to sex, age, current state/UT, and history of death of any acquaintance due to COVID-19; perceived barriers with respect to the type of locality; and health behaviour compliance with respect to age and marital status. Individuals residing in West Bengal at the time of the study, and those having a history of chronic illness, considered themselves more susceptible to COVID-19. Female citizens below the age of 30 years, residing in West Bengal at the time of the study, and those having lost an acquaintance due to COVID-19 were found to perceive the disease to be more severe. Individuals living in semi-urban parts of the country perceived greater amounts of barriers in following preventive behaviours compared to those living in urban areas. Finally, younger citizens (i.e. below 30 years) and those who were unmarried reported to comply to the preventive behaviours more often as compared to older and married groups. However, the respondents did not differ significantly on perceived benefits and self-efficacy across the groups.

Individual Health and the Collective: Results of the Study

Even though there has been a remarkable progress in immunization against the COVID-19 worldwide with the invention and scientific refinement of various vaccines, prevention remains the mainstay in containing the disease, especially in developing nations like India, where there is still a long way to achieve 100% vaccination. Person-to-person transmission being identified as the chief cause of spread of the pandemic, it is crucial to examine human beliefs and behaviours relevant to prevention of the infection. This online survey attempted to assess the preventive behaviours against the spread of COVID-19 based on the HBM constructs in the Indian citizens. In this study, we measured the perceived susceptibility and severity of contracting COVID-19, along with the perceived benefits of, perceived barriers to, and perceived self-efficacy of the respondents in following the prevention recommendations by World Health Organization and Ministry of Health, Government of India. Furthermore, the compliance to these prevention protocols was also evaluated on the basis of the self-reports of the respondents.

The current findings reveal that the perceived susceptibility and severity of the majority of the participants about COVID-19 were relatively low,

Table 1.6 Results of Mann–Whitney U Tests of different components of Health Belief Model (HBM) and compliance to health behaviours across different sociodemographic groups (N = 271)

In each measure, the Male column shows the median with the Mann–Whitney U statistic beneath it; the Female column shows the corresponding median. Values are given as *median / U*.

Category	Perceived Susceptibility		Perceived Severity		Perceived Benefits		Perceived Self-Efficacy		Perceived Barriers		Compliance to Health Behaviours	
	Male	Female	Male	Female	Male	Female	Male	Female	Male	Female	Male	Female
	128 / 8025	141	119 / 6998*	148	129 / 8058	141	132 / 8430	139	134 / 8666	137	136 / 8846	136
Below 30 / Above 30	138 / 7411	132	143 / 6480*	121	141 / 6861	125	139 / 7206	129	132 / 7044	145	144 / 6222*	117
Semi-Urban / Urban	134 / 4444	136	129 / 4266	137	126 / 4127	138	124 / 4062	138	163 / 3470*	131	152 / 3910	133
Other / West Bengal	123 / 7440*	148	125 / 7727*	146	132 / 8586	140	129 / 8249	143	137 / 9078	135	134 / 8970	137
Up to Graduate / Post Graduate	133 / 8811	139	138 / 8924	134	140 / 8608	132	138 / 8874	134	135 / 8982	137	140 / 8675	132
Married / Unmarried	125 / 6438	135	120 / 6058	137	124 / 6366	136	122 / 6227	136	132 / 6944	133	114 / 5622*	140
Absent / Present	129 / 4752*	161	134 / 5713	144	132 / 5392	150	134 / 5667	145	137 / 6025	133	139 / 5540	125

	Did not lose any near one to COVID-19	Lost near one(s) to COVID-19	Did not lose any near one to COVID-19	Lost near one(s) to COVID-19	Did not lose any near one to COVID-19	Lost near one(s) to COVID-19	Did not lose any near one to COVID-19	Lost near one(s) to COVID-19	Did not lose any near one to COVID-19	Lost near one(s) to COVID-19	Did not lose any near one to COVID-19	Lost near one(s) to COVID-19
COVID-19	122	141	119	143	124	141	127	140	138	135	135	136
	6333		6046*		6441		6645		7231		7306	
No H/O COVID-19	133	145	139	128	136	135	138	131	133	144	137	132
	6326		6384		6920		6605		6449		6712	

* p < 0.05

Source: Author/s

suggesting that they did not consider this infection as a threat to their life. In this regard, our results are quite inconsistent with the previous studies which pointed out the individuals perceived higher levels of susceptibility and severity about the disease in India (Hose et al., 2021) as well in other Asian countries like Saudi Arabia (Syed et al., 2021) and Iran (Shahnazi et al., 2020; Mirzaei et al., 2021). However, it critical to consider the time of study in comparing the findings. While the current study was conducted during the end of second wave of the pandemic in India, the previous researchers collected data during early or middle phase of the first wave. Our results indicated that the Indian citizens had become somewhat desensitized to the disease after 1 year of its outbreak, compared to the degree of threat perceived by Indians as well as citizens of other Asian countries during the early phase of the pandemic.

Unlike the perceived threats, the perceived benefits of complying to the preventive behaviours were found to be at a higher level, with the perceived barriers at a relatively lower level. This pattern of benefits outweighing the barriers can be interpreted as a good sign, facilitating the observance of the protective measures. Yehualsh and colleagues (2021) also reported similar findings in Ethiopia where they showed that nearly three-fourth of the respondents (72.0%) agreed with the usefulness of practicing the recommended safety measures to prevent COVID-19 infection, and more than half of participants (55.6%) did not have barriers of COVID-19 infection prevention. Similar patterns were observed in other countries like Poland (Novak et al., 2021) and Iran (Mirazaei et al., 2021). However, a reverse pattern, where benefits of following the protocols were outweighed by the barriers, was also reported by Shahnazi et al. (2020) in the Golestan province of Iran and by Costa (2020) in Brazil. Yet another pattern involving higher levels of both perceived benefits and barriers was observed in India (Hose et al., 2021) and in Saudi Arabia (Syed et al., 2021). Such inconsistencies in results regarding these two HBM constructs across nations and time of study suggest that there may be some other psychological processes and other situational factors influencing the degree to which people around the globe adhere to such beliefs. Future studies must focus on exploring these moderating and mediating factors for a better and holistic understanding of these constructs with respect to the current pandemic. In the current study, the barrier to observing the preventive measures, which was endorsed by a considerable proportion of respondents, was that they had more important concerns in their life than dealing with the pandemic. This can be a result of lower levels of perceived threat itself and can cause potential hindrance against taking adequate protection against the disease by trivializing it. Health authorities and mass media should address this issue to increase more awareness about the pandemic so that the infection does not get trivialized in public perception.

Our results also demonstrated that majority of the respondents perceived their self-efficacy in abiding by the COVID-19 protocols at a relatively higher level. This indicates that the Indian citizens participating in this study believed that they were able to follow the necessary preventive measures adequately. Unlike the other constructs of HBM, this construct has been investigated in relatively fewer studies. Higher levels of self-efficacy were also reported by previous researchers (Nowak et al., 2020; Mirzaei et al., 2021). Shahnazi and colleagues (2020), however, reported considerably low levels of self-efficacy in Iranian population, though they measured this construct by only one general item, while the current study and the other two studies cited employed multiple item measurements of self-efficacy, which is more likely to give a more reliable and integrated evaluation.

The results of our study further showed that majority of the participants adequately followed the disease prevention behaviours except wearing gloves outside home. This indicates that with the outbreak of the disease, although Indian people have become more or less used to wearing masks, the same is not yet true for wearing gloves. Cultural and climatic factors may also be a relevant cause of this non-compliance. Another important finding of this study is that a considerable proportion of Indian citizens are yet to accustom themselves to washing and disinfecting their hands and other personal belongings at regular intervals. Public gatherings are also to be restricted, and it is to be monitored if adequate preventive measures are followed in those gatherings. Government and mass media are to play a pivotal role in creating public awareness, providing them with means and equipment to follow the COVID-19 protocols and maintaining proper surveillance to control the spread of the disease.

In our study, we obtained significant correlation of only one HBM construct, that is perceived severity, with the compliance to prevention measures, suggesting that individuals perceiving COVID-19 to be more severe were more likely to abide by the safety protocols. This is consistent with the theoretical concept of HBM, as well as previous empirical studies (e.g. Nowak et al., 2020; Syed et al., 2021). However, most of the previous studies have also found significant correlations of the other HBM constructs with preventive behaviours, which was not observed in the current study. This is, definitely, a remarkable deviation from the existing literature. One possible reason may be the time of conducting the current study. As Indian population had been somewhat accustomed to the "New Normal" by this time, they might be following the preventive measures by virtue of habit only, without giving much thought to the consequences of not following the measures or the threat imposed by the disease. Future studies are required to delve into this question deeper, employing adequate methodology.

The current study also compared the various HBM constructs and compliance across several sociodemographic groups. Individuals residing in West

Bengal at the time of conducting the study were found to be perceiving themselves to be more susceptible to the infection and believing the infection to be more severe as compared to those residing at other parts of the country. This may be a reflection of the ongoing higher rate of infection in West Bengal at that particular time period. However, this may also be an effect of overrepresentation of participants from this state in the current study. Individuals with history of chronic illness like diabetes, hypertension, and asthma also considered themselves to be more susceptible to the disease compared to otherwise healthy participants. This may be attributed to the awareness programmes emphasizing the fact that individuals with comorbidities are at higher risk for the infection. Female participants were observed to perceive the disease to be more severe than males, which may be suggestive of the innate differences in personality and threat perception across the two sexes. Also, perceived severity of the disease was found to be higher in individuals below 30 years than the older age group. This may be attributed to the greater access of the younger participants to COVID-19-related news, mostly negative. Many youngsters in India were actively engaged in several voluntary services like arranging for hospital admission, oxygen, medicines, and food, among others, for COVID-19 patients, which provided them with a more ground-level information about the gravity of the situation in India, compared to the older citizens, thereby making them perceive the disease to be more severe. Individuals having lost one or more close acquaintances due to COVID-19 had also been impacted negatively by those events of loss, hence becoming more vulnerable to perceive the severity of the outbreak. Greater amounts of barriers to following COVID-19 protocols were reported by respondents from semi-urban regions than those from the urban regions of the country. This may be suggestive of the lack of awareness in the semi-urban regions. As a result, those trying to observe the preventive measures may be feeling quite out of place in absence of a normative observance of those measures. Scarcity in access to the necessary means of preventive measures may also be a potential cause of barriers faced by this group. However, respondents of all the sociodemographic groups were found to perceive comparable levels of benefits of and self-efficacy in abiding by the COVID-19 protocols. Yet another noteworthy finding of our study was that younger and unmarried participants reported of complying to the preventive measures more frequently, compared to the older and married groups.

With the outbreak of a pandemic, where individual health behaviour decisions and compliance is not only relevant to just one's own heath, but also to the health of others, a significant factor might be the degree to which individuals draw personal value from being part of a collective. There is some evidence that the regions of the world that were most successful at containing the pandemic (e.g. countries of the Asian-Pacific rim, see Lowy Institute,

2021; Van Beusekom, 2020) also tend to rank high in collectivism (Hofstede, 2011; Hofstede et al., 2010). In an American sample of students as well, Courtney et al. (2022) demonstrated that under conditions where collectivism was primed (in comparison to individualism), individuals responded to mortality reminders with higher reported intentions to engage in health behaviours helpful for mitigating the spread of the virus. India, being a nation with collectivist principles too, whether health behaviour intentions have been shaped by their cultural values or not need further exploration.

Conclusion

The current study, however, suffers from certain limitations. Though the sample constituted individuals from different parts of the country, the representation was not equal. Moreover, the sample was restricted to semi-urban and urban regions only. Whether the scenario is similar for the rural sector needs examination. The age groups were also not equally distributed. There may be some other methodological concerns of relying only on self-report measures with respect to compliance, because the actual observance might be different from that reported by the respondents due to social desirability bias. Finally, neither of the measures used in this study were developed in India, so some of the items may not be culturally appropriate. Future researchers should attempt to overcome these issues in their studies.

Despite the limitations, our study provides valuable insights in shedding light on the different factors relevant to the health beliefs and compliance to health behaviours, specific to certain sociodemographic groups. Addressing these factors at the policy level by the health authorities as well as by mass media for increasing awareness is expected to result in better observance of COVID-19-safe behaviours in the Indian citizens, thereby facilitating in the containment of the disease.

To conclude, the current study contributes to the previous literature on health behaviours by determining the levels of adherence to different health beliefs and safety protocols by the citizens during later stages of a global pandemic like COVID-19 across different sociodemographic strata in a multicultural nation like India.

References

Alsulaiman, S. A., & Rentner, T. L. (2018). The health belief model and preventive measures: A study of the ministry of health campaign on coronavirus in Saudi Arabia. *Journal of International Crisis and Risk Communication Research, 1*(1), 3.

Champion, V. L. (1984). Instrument development for health belief model constructs. *Advances in nursing science.*

Chan, J. F. W., Yuan, S., Kok, K. H., To, K. K. W., Chu, H., Yang, J., Xing, F., Liu, J., Yip, C. C. Y., Poon, R. W. S., Tsoi, H. W., Lo, S. K. F., Chan, K. H., Poon, V. K. M., Chan, W. M., Ip, J. D., Cai, J. P., Cheng, V. C. C., Chen, H., . . . Yuen, K. Y. (2020). A familial cluster of pneumonia associated with the 2019 novel coronavirus indicating person-to-person transmission: A study of a family cluster. *The Lancet, 395*(10223), 514–523.

Costa, M. F. (2020). Health belief model for coronavirus infection risk determinants. *Revista de Saúde Pública, 54.*

Courtney, E. P., Felig, R. N., & Goldenberg, J. L. (2022). Together we can slow the spread of COVID-19: The interactive effects of priming collectivism and mortality salience on virus-related health behaviour intentions. *British Journal of Social Psychology, 61*(1), 410–431.

Friedman, H. S., & Kern, M. L. (2014). Personality, well-being, and health. *Annual Review of Psychology, 65,* 719–742.

Glanz, K., Rimer, B. K., & Viswanath, K. (Eds.). (2008). *Health behavior and health education: Theory, research, and practice.* John Wiley & Sons.

Grodner, M. (1991). Using the health belief model for bulimia prevention. *Journal of American College Health, 40*(3), 107–112.

Grosser, L. R. (1982). Health belief model aids understanding of patient behavior. *AORN Journal, 35*(6), 1056–1059.

Hofstede, G. (2011). *Culture's consequences: Comparing values, behaviors, institutions, and organizations across nations.* Sage Publications.

Hofstede, G., Hofstede, G. J., & Minkov, M. (2010). *Cultures and organizations: Software of the mind* (Revised and expanded 3rd ed.). McGraw-Hill.

Hurley, A. C. (1990). The health belief model: Evaluation of a diabetes scale. *The Diabetes Educator, 16*(1), 44–48.

Jose, R., Narendran, M., Bindu, A., Beevi, N., Manju, L., & Benny, P. V. (2021). Public perception and preparedness for the pandemic COVID-19: A health belief model approach. *Clinical Epidemiology and Global Health, 9,* 41–46.

Kamran, A., Isazadehfar, K., Pirzadeh, A., Azgomi, R. N. D., & Heydari, H. (2020). *Risk perception and adherence to preventive behaviors by the public amid COVID-19 pandemic; a community-based study applying the health belief model.* https://scholar.google.com/citations?view_op=view_citation&hl=en&user=eAN qUNYAAAAJ&citation_for_view=eANqUNYAAAAJ:M3NEmzRMIkIC

Lowy Institute. (2021). *COVID performance index: Deconstructing pandemic responses.* https://interactives.lowyinstitute.org/features/covidperformance/#r egion

Ministry of Health. (2021, November 21). *COVID-19 INDIA as on November 21, 2021.* www.mohfw.gov.in

Mirzaei, A., Kazembeigi, F., Kakaei, H., Jalilian, M., Mazloomi, S., & Nourmoradi, H. (2021). Application of health belief model to predict COVID-19-preventive behaviors among a sample of Iranian adult population. *Journal of Education and Health Promotion, 10.*

Nowak, B., Brzóska, P., Piotrowski, J., Sedikides, C., Żemojtel-Piotrowska, M., & Jonason, P. K. (2020). Adaptive and maladaptive behavior during the

COVID-19 pandemic: The roles of dark triad traits, collective narcissism, and health beliefs. *Personality and Individual Differences, 167*, 110232.

Person, B., Sy, F., Holton, K., Govert, B., & Liang, A. (2004). Fear and stigma: The epidemic within the SARS outbreak. *Emerging Infectious Diseases, 10*(2), 358.

Rosenstock, I. M. (1974). The health belief model and preventive health behavior. *Health Education Monographs, 2*(4), 354–386.

Rosenstock, I. M., Strecher, V. J., & Becker, M. H. (1988). Social learning theory and the health belief model. *Health Education Quarterly, 15*(2), 175–183.

Sayegh, P., & Knight, B. G. (2013). Cross-cultural differences in dementia: The sociocultural health belief model. *International Psychogeriatrics, 25*(4), 517–530.

Shahnazi, H., Ahmadi-Livani, M., Pahlavanzadeh, B., Rajabi, A., Hamrah, M. S., & Charkazi, A. (2020). Assessing preventive health behaviors from COVID-19: A cross sectional study with health belief model in Golestan Province, Northern of Iran. *Infectious Diseases of Poverty, 9*(1), 1–9.

Sjödin, H., Wilder-Smith, A., Osman, S., Farooq, Z., & Rocklöv, J. (2020). Only strict quarantine measures can curb the Coronavirus disease (COVID-19) outbreak in Italy, 2020. *Eurosurveillance, 25*(13), 2000280.

Syed, M. H., Meraya, A. M., Yasmeen, A., Albarraq, A. A., Alqahtani, S. S., Syed, N. K. A., Algarni, M. A., & Alam, N. (2021). Application of the health belief model to assess community preventive practices against COVID-19 in Saudi Arabia. *Saudi Pharmaceutical Journal, 29*(11).

Van Beusekom, M. (2020). *New tool ranks COVID-19 responses of 19 hard-hit nations.* Center for Infectious Disease Research and Policy. www.cidrap.umn.edu/newsperspective/2020/10/new-tool-ranks-covid-19-responses-19-hard-hit-nations

Wilder-Smith, A., & Freedman, D. O. (2020). Isolation, quarantine, social distancing and community containment: Pivotal role for old-style public health measures in the novel Coronavirus (2019-nCoV) outbreak. *Journal of Travel Medicine, 27*.

Wilson, A. R., Brega, A. G., Thomas, J. F., Henderson, W. G., Lind, K. E., Braun, P. A., Batliner, T. S., & Albino, J. (2018). Validity of measures assessing oral health beliefs of American Indian parents. *Journal of Racial and Ethnic Health Disparities, 5*(6), 1254–1263.

Yehualashet, S., Asefa, K. K., Mekonnen, A. G., Gemeda, B. N., Shiferaw, W. S., Aynalem, Y. A., Bilchut, A. H., Derseh, B. T., Mekuria, A. D., Mekonnen, W. N., Meseret, W. A., Tegegnework, S. S., & Abosetegn, A. E. (2021). Predictors of adherence to COVID-19 prevention measure among communities in North Shoa Zone, Ethiopia based on health belief model: A cross-sectional study. *PLoS One, 16*(1), e0246006.

2 Unveiling Stigma

Exploring Mental Health Literacy in the Time of COVID-19 Pandemic

Avisikta Basu and Tilottama Mukherjee

Introduction

The world has seen a wave of changes in the past 2 years while being a victim on one hand and a survivor on the other. Mental Health or mental illness and related issues have appeared a number of times as a part of the front-page discussion, globally, off late. Some of the recent research indicates that the ongoing COVID-19 pandemic may have led to a major deterioration in people's Mental Health (MH), because of the increase in social isolation and loneliness (Holmes et al., 2020; Pierce et al., 2020).

On the other hand, during the past 3 years of the COVID-19 pandemic, Mental Health awareness has been brought into light through different formal and informal discussions, which mostly limited to the month of October, earlier, now seem to be buzzing around year long. Recently, the world has seen a global rise in the number of cases related to Mental Health and general well-being. Current studies show that Mental Health is worsening among all age groups, and stigma plays one of the biggest contributing role in it. Stigma around Mental Health and lack of access to the necessary care are driving many people away from getting the care that they need. A study conducted in 2021 shows that education about neurodegenerative disorders is urgently needed on social media to address COVID-19-related stigma. And if stigmatising discourse on dementia is shared through different media and consumed among the public, it was observed to have public health implications as a result.

It can be said that the stigma and help-seeking tend to have a bidirectional relationship with each other. The stigmatisation leads to disparities in the availability of help and vice versa. Ben-Porath (2002) reported in their study that individuals with a mental illness who were seeking help were seen more negatively than those individuals with only a mental illness.

Goffman defined stigma as an attribute that is deeply discrediting. On the other hand, Mental Health stigma includes the perception that people with mental illness are flawed and or weak in nature.

DOI: 10.4324/9781003348429-2

The question arises what are the factors existing in the society, which contribute to the prevailing Mental Health stigma?

Corrigan (2004) in his work indicated that mental illness was a "two-edged sword" (p. 403). "On one side was psychological distress that debilitated a person from normal and optimal functioning. On the other side was stigma that hindered an individual from taking necessary action to alleviate psychological distress" (Corrigan, 2004). There are different kinds of existing Mental Health stigmas. For example in one research, it has been shown that in the North East side of the country of India, it is believed that all mental illnesses are alike. The cause is presumed to be a single shock, sexual starvation, result of "Heat," or of possession. As per the same research, interestingly, "Most of the Misconception" is present in the educated and sophisticated section of the society.

Perhaps an extension of the concept of Mental Health stigma is help-seeking, which involves obtaining help in terms of understanding, the advice, support in response to a problem, or a distressing experience. Although it could be of two types, formal and informal, here the focus is on formal help-seeking from a professional source.

During 2020, when the global pandemic due to COVID-19 virus had set in, it had an immense negative impact on the area of Mental Health. During this period, the data from all over the world show that concerns about Mental Health and substance use have grown, including concerns about suicidal ideation. In the KIFF study which was conducted in January 2021, 41% of adults reported having symptoms of anxiety and/or depressive disorder, a share that has been largely stable since spring 2020. In another survey from June 2020, 13% of adults reported new or an increase in the substance use due to COVID-19 virus-related stress, and 11% of adults reported thoughts of suicide in the past 30 days.

Lack of discussion and the recognition of mental illness as well as Mental Health are identified as some of the major reasons why the ever-existing stigmas are there, but the picture seems to have changed during the pandemic, that is different articles shed light on this pertinent factor during the pandemic. Moreover, as the perceived need and different attitudinal barriers were found to be the reasons why there exist the barriers to MH treatment (Andrade et al., 2014; Mojtabai et al., 2011), it could be conceptualised that improving MH literacy and a reduction in the stigma may help overcome these barriers and increase the access and use of necessary MH services when needed. As per Corrigan (2000) "This is also important for reducing the negative consequences of MH stigma, including but not limited to one's self-esteem, social opportunities, as well as work and living opportunities."

During this phase, a number of initiatives were being taken to change the negative attitude towards it. For example the Government of India has initiated a number of programmes like the *National Mental Health Program (NMHP)* and *District Mental Health Program (DMHP)*. But the question remains, do this discussion, multiple articles, and awareness programmes really contribute to making any change in the deep-rooted stigma around it (negative perception of mental illness as well as the mentally ill) or the necessary professional help-seeking?

Job loss, economic downfall, closure of colleges and universities, and work from home culture, all of these, had adverse effects on the current Mental Health of the population in concern, but did that actually have an impact on help-seeking further?

Quoting a recent article,

> My interactions with the community have often revealed that people do not want to consult a psychiatrist or visit a Mental Health facility because of the social stigma associated with the same. Discussion of Mental Health issues on news and social media often does not help the majority of the Indian population due to a lack of education as well as language gaps, given that most of such coverage takes place in English.
>
> Dr Sarkar, COVID-19 has exacerbated India's hidden Mental Health pandemic, *Indiabioscience.org*

The picture before pandemic shows a number of evidences where the stigma stands tall between the people who need help and the availability of formal help. In a study by R. C. Kessler et al. (2001), it was found that age is a determining factor in case of help-seeking, and this was found to be less in case of young adults.

In another research by Bolder and Fallon (1995), it was observed that some types of problems are more likely to prompt help-seeking behaviour than others, and different sources of help are deemed more appropriate for particular types of problems. For example the study showed that relationship problems are often discussed with friends, personal problems with the parents, and educational problems are more likely to be taken to the teachers. For this research concerned, some of the factors were taken into consideration using previous literature, which were emotional intelligence, perceived social support, and resilience.

In a study by Kondrat et al. (2018), they explored whether perceived social support works as a mediator between the impact of experienced discrimination and Mental Health. We also test the moderating hypotheses as a way to determine if past research on the role of perceived social support is a better model than the mediating model. They used data from a subset of 32 Canadian Community Health Survey-Mental Health. The results suggest that perceived social support mediates the relationship between the impact of experienced or perceived discrimination and Mental Health.

Resilience, on the other hand, is considered as an asset to human existence. In common words, it is the ability to bounce back after one has encountered a stressor. One common definition of resilience is "multi-dimensional characteristic that varies with context, time, age, gender and cultural origin, as well as within an individual subject to different life circumstances." Resilience can be seen from different lights of hardiness, benefit finding, thriving, etc. These all operate separately or in combination in order to make the person work with resilience.

Emotional intelligence which is conceptualised as one's ability to assess, understand, and control others' and one's own emotion perhaps is a part of most of the researches at present. A person's understanding of own emotion involves the understanding of current state of Mental Health as well as this involves one's emotional expression. Whether a person's tendency and/or ability to perceive the status of mental well-being and further seeking help for it could be hypothesised as a journey and EQ is a mediating factor there.

In the present chapter, an attempt is made to explore the persisting Mental Health stigma and its association with the aforementioned construct from a quantitative perspective.

Methods

Sampling method – Sampling was done using Non probability, Purposive method.

Participants were taken in three groups, with the age ranging from 18 to 45 years. The first group comprised young adults (18–26 years), second group comprised late adults (27–35 years), and third group (36–45 years) had both males and females. They were fluent in English, well acquainted with technology, and willing to participate in the study. The age difference was found to be significant with a t value of 22.83 (significant at 0.00 level).

Inclusion criteria were: (i) age between 18 and 45 years; (ii) currently not undergoing or have not undergone any psychiatric treatment; (iii) can read, write, and understand English.

Exclusion criterion was: people who had psychiatric educational background.

Informed consent was obtained from participants, and the study design did not contain any aspects needing ethical evaluation.

Measures

1. *The CAMIS (Community Attitude Towards Mentally Ill Scale)* was developed in 1979 by Martin Taylor and Michael Dear and is used to assess the attitude towards mental illness and mentally ill of the community population. CAMI contains 40 statements which claim mental illness and are rated on a five-degree Likert-scale (CAMI Scale, 2017b). The scale has a good construct and criterion validity, and reliability of different subscales are found as follows: Authoritarianism .68, Benevolence .76, Social Restrictiveness .80, and Community Mental Health Ideology .88.

2. *Attitude Towards Seeking Professional Help – Short Form (ATSPH-SF)*

   This Scale was developed on an established Self Report Measure of named 'Attitude Towards Seeking Mental Health Care' (Fisher & Turner, 1970). Fischer and Farina (1995) developed a shortened version with college students. The shortened version of ATSPH was developed by retaining the 14 original items possessing the largest item-total score correlations (found in Fischer & Turner, 1970). One of these factors included 10 items, which were retained to produce a unidimensional measure of treatment attitudes. The short form uses the same response format as the original measure and a four-point Likert type scale (0 = "Disagree" to 3 = "Agree") but has several minor rewordings to represent contemporary terminology (Fischer & Farina, 1995).

   The short version has demonstrated internal consistency ranging from 0.82 to 0.84 (Fischer & Farina, 1995; Komiya et al., 2000; Miville & Constantine, 2006), one month test–retest reliability of 0.80, and a correlation of 0.87 with the longer scale (Fischer & Farina, 1995), among samples of college students.

3. *The Emotional Intelligence Scale* by Hyde et al. (2002) is used to measure the emotional intelligence from an ability perspective of the participants through different subscales. It contains 34 items. The obtainable score ranges from 34 to 170, where higher score indicates higher level of emotional intelligence.

4. *The MPSSS (Multidimensional Perceived Social Support Scale)* was developed by Zimet et al. (1988) and used to measure the current perceived social support of the participants of both the age groups. The MSPSS is a brief, easy-to-administer self-report questionnaire which contains 12 items rated on a seven-point Likert-type scale, with scores ranging from "very strongly disagree" (1) to "very strongly agree" (7). It is a reliable and valid measure to assess the perceived social support.

5. *The Resilience Scale* by Wagnild and Young (1993)—The 25-item Resilience Scale (Wagnild & Young, 1993) measures the degree of

individual resilience through five components: equanimity, perseverance, self-reliance, meaningfulness, and existential aloneness. The scoring ranges from 1 to 7, Strongly disagree to strongly agree. According to previous studies, resilience measured by the RS has a positive correlation with life satisfaction, self-esteem, self-rated health, self-actualisation, stress management, and social support, and a negative correlation with depressive symptoms and anxiety (Abiola & Udofia, 2011; Heilemann et al., 2003; Humphreys, 2003; Nishi et al., 2010; Wagnild, 2009; Wagnild & Young, 1993).

Analyses

Scores were distributed normally in the population, and parametric statistics were used for the analyses. Analysis of Variance (ANOVA), t-test, Pearson Product Moment Correlation, and Multiple Regression were used.

Results

Tables 2.1 to 2.6 here show the result of the analyses.

Table 2.1 Sociodemographic details

Mean Age	
YA:LA: EML	21.83: 28.63: 39.57
Sex	
Males: Females	52: 48
Education	
Graduate: Postgraduate	80: 20
Marital STATUS	
Married: Unmarried	61: 39
Family Type	
Nuclear: Joint	78:22
Residence	
Urban: Suburban	67: 33

Source: Author/s

Table 2.2 Findings of the Analysis of Variance (ANOVA) amongst different age groups

Variables	*F Value*
ATSPH	1.53
CAMIS	
Authoritarianism	6.68*
Benevolence	38.68*
Social Restrictedness	3.85*

(*Continued*)

Table 2.2 (Continued)

Variables	F Value
Community Mental Health Ideology	6.08*
Emotional Intelligence	37.84*
Perceived Social Support	6.57*
Family	2.26
Friends	1.44
Significant Other	5.20
Resilience	8.32*

*Significant at 0.05 level of significance.

Source: Author/s

Table 2.3 Findings of the t-test between the males and the females

	t-Value
ATSPH	−1.81
CAMIS	
Authoritarianism	2.114
Benevolence	2.77*
Social Restrictedness	−0.49*
Community Mental Health Ideology	−0.516
Emotional Intelligence	1.064
Perceived Social Support	3.2
Family	1.98
Friends	3.1
Significant Other	−0.48
Resilience	−0.006

Source: Author/s

Discussion

The study primarily aims to assess the current status of Mental Health Literacy in India during the pandemic through the lens of age and sex. To explore and understand this, the variables that were taken into considerations were attitude towards seeking help, attitude towards mental illness, emotional intelligence, perceived social support, and resilience.

The scores obtained through the statistical analysis indicate that there exists a significant difference in terms of the attitude towards mental illness (Table 2.1). Young adults have scored higher in domains which are positively correlated with stigma and late adults – that is the next age group – has obtained higher scores on domains which are negatively correlated with stigma. Now, the domains as assessed by CAMIS mentioned earlier in the chapter are authoritarianism that reflects a view of the mentally ill as an

Table 2.4 Findings of the correlations

	ATSPH	EI	AU	BE	SOC	COMM	FAM	FR	SO	PSS	Resilience
ATSPH	1	0.091	0.977	0.192*	-0.037	-.123				-0.096	0.192*
EI		1	-0.256*	0.318*	-0.062	0.209*				-0.226	0.293*
Authoritarianism			1				0.080	0.015	0.068	0.107	-0.210*
Benevolence				1			-0.083	-0.040	-0.061	-0.171	
Social Restrictedness					1		0.082	-0.091	-0.083	0.198	
Community Mental Health Ideology						1	0.004	-0.047	0.098	0.425	
Family							1				
Friends								1			
Significant Others									1		
PSS										1	-0.101
Resilience											1

* Significant at 0.05 level of significance.

Source: Author/s

Table 2.5 Significant findings of regression analysis

Criterion	Predictor	r-Square
Benevolence	Emotional intelligence	0.118*
ATSPH	Benevolence	0.002
ATSPH	Resilience	0.039*
Community Mental Health ideology	Emotional intelligence	0.035*

* Significant at 0.05 level

Source: Author/s

Table 2.6 Graph showing the mean values obtained by each group in different scales

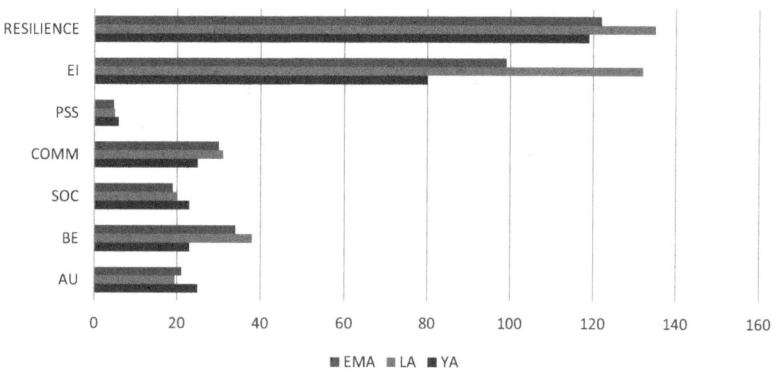

Scores obtained on different Scales with significant difference

Source: Author/s

inferior class than the rest, requiring coercive handling; benevolence that is a paternalistic as well as sympathetic view of patients based on humanistic principles; Mental Health ideology, a medical model that views mental illness similar to any other illness; and social restrictiveness that means viewing the mentally ill as a threat to the society. Hence, it indicates that with aging, the perception towards mental illness changes, and the stigma around it decreases although from late adulthood to early middle age, it does not vary significantly. To elaborate on this, it can be said that the result can be attributed to the fact that the change of developmental tasks and increased responsibility taking and exposure to the world lead to less stigmatised attitude, and an acceptance of the mental illness and mentally ill also takes place. In aging research, the socio-emotional selectivity theory similarly suggests divergent effects of aging on cognitive and emotional functions: whereas cognitive abilities decline, affective functions are considered to stay intact or even increase with old age.

Individuals who perceive the future as long will invest in emotionally taxing activities (caring for social desirability, subsiding own emotions just to be liked and accepted by a broader space, i.e. not just peers but society in general) – I desire and need to be liked and accepted and in a way to adjust better in social and occupational life than in the personal life by caring for own health situations that include the mental and physical health. In other words, when the future is constrained and time is perceived to be limited, the importance of emotion-related goals start growing. Under such temporal conditions, individuals tend to prioritise their emotional satisfaction over the desire of exploration and gathering information from that. People are motivated to invest in emotionally meaningful experiences that will provide more immediate payoffs. This prioritises close relationships and emotionally meaningful interactions. Older adults maintain their most meaningful, core relationships and let go of less satisfying, peripheral social partners. Similarly, when asked to imagine they have a half hour of free time, older adults prefer to spend time with a close social partner rather than a novel one, whereas younger adults do not show this preference. With these, the desire to maintain social desirability also lessens which contributes to the decrease in stigma. The results also show a significant drop in the perceived social support from young adults to late adults. There have been a number of researches on different cultural contexts related to the age being the mediator of PSS. The results show that the younger groups emotionally benefit from using both explicit and implicit support, whereas the older adults emotionally benefit from using implicit support more where they do not have to seek the support by asking for it directly. Young people seek and receive more social support from their family and or friends (Levitt et al., 1993), and any stress or distress leads to seeking help from their social circle available (Parker & Parrott, 1995), and self-disclosure with friends, not family, is negatively associated with their feelings of loneliness (Franzoi & Davis, 1985). So, in a way, older people rely more on the coping skills that they carry within themselves along with time; in reference to the social selectivity theory also, they restrict themselves from looking for more social support available, and mostly are content with the strength that they carry within themselves, which is not reflected explicitly. Another perspective that can be added to it is the PGI model or the concept of personal growth initiative. PGI is observed to work as a predictor of self stigma and eventually the tendency to seek help for the MH issues (Seidman et al., 2022). PGI, that is "a person's ability to identify areas for change and initiate growth" plays a role in decision-making which includes the decision to seek treatment as well, so one's willingness to grow and develop into a better person with age could also be identified here in case of the present research to be responsible for reduced stigma in the older group.

Further understanding can come from the perspective that time and education in general can contribute to the change in stigma. So the findings actually support the work of Losada et al. (2012) and a very popular research of the decade, *Time to Change* (2015), suggesting that as an individual ages they become more informed about and accepting of those who differ from them. Similar research findings also suggested that the people of older group are more willing to accept the need for different Mental Health care and eventually increased contact with people with mental illness, which is reflected in the items under benevolence and Mental Health ideology scale of CAMI which are indicative of less stigmatised attitude (Henderson et al., 2020). In line with the meta-analyses conducted by Corrigan et al. (2012), Grifths et al. (2014) found that those in the 40 years and over age group are more likely to have had sustained contact with an individual with a Mental Health diagnosis, potentially reducing stigmatised attitudes. This also supports findings of a research by Jorm and Wright (2008) who report that young people are more inclined to view mental illness as a personal failure or weakness rather than a valid health problem. During the young age, the coping strategies, self-esteem, and sensitivity all are in a developing stage, which actually grow and further gets revised repeatedly with more social exposure. But there are researches which show it is not a continuous process that a person's overall perception keeps changing every moment (Wolska & Pietrulewicz, 2008), which is also observed in the present study that shows no significant difference in any of the domains of CAMIS between late adults and early middle-aged adults.

Now, that scores in ATSPPH do not differ significantly with different age groups is another notable observation of this study. The previous, yet a very latest, research indicates otherwise, as per a research done by Kawabata et al. (2022), high public stigma leads to lower intent or tendency to seek Mental Health treatment or professional help through an indirect pathway of one's self-stigma. The different findings of the present research can be analysed if the concept or factors related to seeking help or seeking treatment can be understood. Early researches suggest that help-seeking is the process of actively seeking out and utilising social relationships, either formal or informal, to help with personal problems. Unlike many other social transactional processes, the objective in help-seeking is intensely personal. Help-seeking lies on the contrary at the nexus of the personal and interpersonal. Consequently, factors that affect both these domains are relevant, but those that operate at their intersection are especially pertinent. The initial stage is personal where there is an effect of the awareness of the personal domain in relation to Mental Health problems, the ability to articulate or express this personal domain to others, and willingness to disclose to these people which

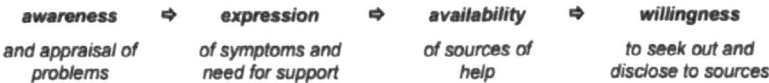

Figure 2.1 Model of Help-Seeking (Rickwood et al. 2005)

Source: Author/s

comes in the second stage is intensely interpersonal. The following process model of help-seeking guided in the research design of help-seeking was conceptualised as a process whereby the personal becomes increasingly interpersonal. So although the attitude towards mental illness is significantly different while filling up the questionnaire that asks, "If I believed I was having a mental breakdown, my first inclination would be to get professional attention" or "I might want to have psychological counselling in the future," participants from all the three groups have rated higher. This can be explained by the social desirability and current global conditions during COVID-19 pandemic. Over social, printing and electronic media, various campaigning have been made to emphasise the need to seek professional help when needed and focussing on the medical model more (which presents mental illness as any other physical illness).

The groups differ significantly with respect to emotional intelligence (EI) and resilience. In the current study, emotional intelligence was found to increase gradually with age. There is a significant difference between the EI of young and late adults but not between late and early middle-aged adults. This is supported by the research evidences that age is directly correlated with a higher EI. Life experiences are an important contributory factor in the development of EI (Birol et al., 2009). As individuals mature, they become more sensitive to the feelings of others, to a large extent. However, the gradual change in empathy with age is often minimum, which explains the not significant change in EI between the late adults and early middle-aged adults (Lorenzo, 2008). Resilience on the other hand seems to have increased significantly in case of late adults but decreased in the next age group, that is early middle aged adults. Resilience is often determined by factors like respect, responsibility, and values, and all of these tend to grow with the passing of time as a person passes through different ages, resulting in a change in the person's resilient self as well. Resilience may change over time as a function of development and one's interaction with the environment (e.g. Kim-Cohen & Turkewitz, 2012, p. 92). For example high maternal care and protection may be resilience-enhancing during one's infancy period but may interfere with individuation during adolescence or young adulthood. When we think about resilience as a process, then we are talking about an organism that is actively interacting with an environment.

So with aging, when the person is in the early ages, that is young adulthood along with the biological caregiver, the exposure and interaction with the environment are less and with time they might increase later which is observed in the late adults where, developmentally speaking, a person is entering a new world where another bond is being formed that is starting a family, which is beyond the biological bond he/she was carrying. Along with that, the contribution of entering into the professional world, financial independence, could not be ignored.

Results show that there are significant differences in terms of the attitude towards mental illness between male and female of different age groups (Table 2.2). A look at most of the previous researches suggests that girls and women are more likely to seek help than boys and men. This varies according to the source of help and type of the problem, but overall results have suggested previously that females are more likely to seek out other people for support and advice for Mental Health problems (Boldero & Fallon, 1995; Rickwood & Braithwaite, 1994). In contrast, a male is more likely to rely on himself than to seek help from other people and is also more likely to avoid recognition or deny the presence of a problem in the first place (Offer et al., 1991). *Time to Change* (2015) reports a noticeable difference when examining attitudes from a perspective of social construct, gender; it shows that females are consistently reported to be more understanding, less fearful, and less likely to exclude those with mental illness, but that does not corroborate with the other findings of this study in case of emotional intelligence as no significant difference is observed with respect to sex findings in CAMIS scale, that is a significant difference in case of benevolence and authoritarianism, as it is already mentioned, these two domains are negatively correlated with each other. Females are found to be on the higher side of benevolence subscale and males scored higher on the authoritarianism domain. This again supports the findings that females are more empathetic and accepting towards not only the concept of mental illness but also towards the Mental Health care system as a whole and the need for providing support to the mentally ill people. Although literature shows females are more prone to help-seeking in the current research, the degree of difference between the scores from the sex perspective is not statistically significant.

The correlation findings (Table 2.4) suggest that ATSPH holds a positive correlation with emotional intelligence and the Benevolence Scale of CAMIS. The result indicates that higher a person's emotional intelligence is and the more benevolent attitude a person has towards the people with mental illness, the more prone he is to seek professional help. So the less stigmatised a person is attitude of his is more sympathetic with better understanding of the concept of mental illness and person suffering from any mental illness. and as this will result in the perception of mental illness as well as the treatment for it as a normal and necessary step, the tendency to seek help in case of their own need is higher also.

Higher score on emotional intelligence scale also indicates one's ability to become more empathetic and aware about emotional need and manage them, which also is related positively with help-seeking attitude. Theories of help-seeking suggest that the lack of emotional competence is one potential barrier to seeking help. There are two possible ways that emotional intelligence could have an impact on help-seeking. It is possible that people with low emotional intelligence have the highest intention to seek help for their emotional problems because they feel less capable of handling those emotions on their own. Conversely, it is also possible that people with low emotional competence are the least likely to seek help because they lack some of the skills required to so effectively. Low emotional intelligence might be thought to be associated with less willingness to seek help. Thus, the positive relationship of EI and benevolence also explains its positive correlation with Community Mental Health ideology. Perceived social support (PSS), which is defined as how much a person feels supported, cared for, and loved by the network around him, is observed to have a significant negative correlation with benevolence. It can be explained that the more the person feels safe, accepted, and sure of getting the necessary support in case of any stress, the less the person feels empathetic and identifies with people with any mental illness, and as a result is more rigid and less accepting of the 'Others'. As the literature indicates, especially in crisis times or emotional strain occasions, it is normal that individuals need to have endurance natural helpers like family members, friends, and other close environment. Similarly, in the case of less perceived social support, the empathetic understanding and positive Mental Health ideology develops resulting from a personal need or craving of being supported. On the other hand, its positive correlation with social restrictiveness domain could be viewed from the perspective that the more the person feels connected with the group he belongs to, the more prominent the discrimination of people with mental illness as being the "other group" becomes. This is directly related to the concept of stigma: the more of social restrictedness that a person possesses the higher will be the perceived difference between a mentally healthy and unhealthy person. This will lead to further discrimination.

Findings of linear regression (Table 2.4) show that the tendencies of seeking professional psychological help can be predicted by benevolence, that is a sympathetic attitude towards mental illness as well as towards people with mental illness and resilience. It can be explained this way that if a person sees mental illness from an objective perspective and just as a problem and people with mental illness as sufferers, that definitely results in less stigma or discrimination towards mental illness. Eventually that helps to develop an attitude that is reflected in some items of ATSPH like "A person with an emotional problem is not likely to solve it alone; he or she is likely to solve it with professional help." Resilience, as has been argued by different literatures, is a construct that helps a person to bounce back, keeping the hope alive; this also suggests that the more resilient a person would be, the more he will see the disorder from the medical perspective and would seek formal help to come out of it. Another criterion that has been used in the regression analysis was Community Mental Health Ideology of CAMIS, and findings show that it is predicted by one's emotional intelligence. Now emotional intelligence or one's competence to understand, assess, and respond to one's own and others' emotional adequately is thought to play a role in whether a person will have an accepting attitude towards the Mental Health problem and whether he would see it in a positive light. So Mental Health stigma can be predicted by one's emotional competence or, in other words, emotional maturity which is assessed by his EQ. The more a person is aware of the emotional state of self and others, the less is the rigidity regarding the opinions and perceptions of people with mental illness. Most people who seek help for a Mental Health problem do so from a general physician instead of Mental Health professional (Parslow & Jorm, 2000). Likewise, the findings also show that another component of community's attitude towards mental illness which is benevolence can also be predicted by emotional intelligence, so it is indicated that EI is not just associated with benevolence positively but also is able to predict it, and a change brought in one's EI can affect the benevolent attitude towards the concept of mental illness.

Conclusion

Summarising all of the aforementioned findings, it could be said that the research conducted in the COVID-19 pandemic situation shows that Mental Health stigma is quite prevalent in current Indian society across different age groups. The initial surge of COVID-19 cases followed by a hike in Mental Health problems as well as changes in the number and kind of the awareness programmes did not bring a significant change in the deep-rooted Mental Health stigmas. The stigma is observed to change gradually with age, but the difference with the increase of age becomes less significant after a period of time. Males and females also differ in terms of their attitude towards Mental illness and their tendencies of help-seeking. Along with that, factors like emotional intelligence play an important and integral part of not just people's attitude towards the ill and illness but also are a determining factor in case of their attitude to seek professional help when necessary.

Limitations of the present research and suggestions for further research

The research has explored the Mental Health literacy from a quantitative perspective, identifying the current status of it. Due to the ongoing pandemic and other restrictions of collecting and accessing the necessary information, detailed further qualitative analysis could not be done. Further research could explore other variables apart from the sociodemographic ones and the status in different minority populations as well. A qualitative approach to look into the causal and explanatory aspects behind such results would be beneficial to the field of Mental Health.

References

Abiola, T., & Udofia, O. (2011). Psychometric assessment of the Wagnild and Young's resilience scale in Kano, Nigeria. *BMC Research Notes, 4*(1), 1–5.

Aguon, C. T., & Kawabata, Y. (2022). Examining mental health stigma on Guam: A serial mediation model. *Asian American Journal of Psychology*. Advance online publication. https://doi.org/10.1037/aap0000286

Andrade, L. H., Alonso, J., Mneimneh, Z., Wells, J. E., Al-Hamzawi, A., Borges, G., ... & Kessler, R. C. (2014). Barriers to mental health treatment: results from the WHO World Mental Health surveys. *Psychological medicine, 44*(6), 1303–1317.

Ben-Porath, D. D. (2002). Stigmatization of individuals who receive psychotherapy: An interaction between help-seeking behavior and the presence of depression. *Journal of Social and Clinical Psychology, 21*(4), 400–413.

Birol, C., Atamtürk, H., Silman, F., & Şensoy, Ş. (2009). Analysis of the emotional intelligenge level of teachers. *Procedia-Social and Behavioral Sciences, 1*(1), 2606–2614.

Boldero, J., & Fallon, B. (1995). Adolescent help-seeking: What do they get help for and from whom? *Journal of Adolescence, 18*(2), 193–209.

Corrigan, P. W. (2000). Mental health stigma as social attribution: Implications for research methods and attitude change. *Clinical Psychology: Science and Practice, 7*(1), 48.

Corrigan, P. W. (2004). How stigma interferes with mental health care. *American Psychologist, 59*(7), 614.

Corrigan, P. W., Morris, S. B., Michaels, P. J., Rafacz, J. D., & Rüsch, N. (2012). Challenging the public stigma of mental illness: A meta-analysis of outcome studies. *Psychiatric Services, 63*(10), 963–973.

Dear, M.J., and Taylor, S.M. *Community Attitudes Toward Neighbourhood Public Facilities*. Report submitted to Social Science and Humanities Research Council of Canada, Ottawa, September 1979.

Fariselli, L., Ghini, M., & Freedman, J. (2008). Age and emotional intelligence. *Six Seconds: The Emotional Intelligence Network*, 1–10.

Fisher, E., & Farina, A. (1995). Attitudes toward seeking professional psychological help: Development and research utility of an attitude scale. *Journal of College Student Development, 36*, 368–373.

Fischer, E. H., & Turner, J. L. (1970). Orientations to seeking professional help: Development and research utility of an attitude scale. *Journal of Consulting and Clinical Psychology, 35*, 79–90.

Franzoi, S. L., & Davis, M. H. (1985). Adolescent self-disclosure and loneliness: private self-consciousness and parental influences. *Journal of Personality and Social Psychology, 48*(3), 768.

González-Torres, M. A., Oraa, R., Arístegui, M., Fernández-Rivas, A., & Guimon, J. (2007). Stigma and discrimination towards people with schizophrenia and their family members. *Social Psychiatry and Psychiatric Epidemiology, 42*(1), 14–23.

Griffiths, K. M., Carron-Arthur, B., Parsons, A., & Reid, R. (2014). Effectiveness of programs for reducing the stigma associated with mental disorders. A meta-analysis of randomized controlled trials. *World psychiatry, 13*(2), 161–175.

Heilemann, M. V., Lee, K., & Kury, F. S. (2003). Psychometric properties of the Spanish version of the Resilience Scale. *Journal of nursing measurement, 11*(1), 61–72.

Henderson, C., Potts, L., & Robinson, E. J. (2020). Mental illness stigma after a decade of Time to Change England: inequalities as targets for further improvement. *European journal of public health, 30*(3), 497–503.

Holmes, E. A., O'Connor, R. C., Perry, V. H., Tracey, I., Wessely, S., Arseneault, L., Ballard, C. G., Christensen, H., Cohen Silver, R., Everall, I., Ford, T., John, A., Kabir, T., King, K., Madan, I., Michie, S., Przybylski, A. K., Shafran, R., Sweeney, A., . . . Bullmore, E. (2020). Multidisciplinary research priorities for the COVID-19 pandemic: A call for action for mental health science. *The Lancet Psychiatry, 7*(6), 547–560.

Humphreys, J. (2003). Resilience in sheltered battered women. *Issues in mental health nursing, 24*(2), 137–152.

Hyde, A., Pethe, S., & Dhar, U. (2001). *Emotional intelligence scale: Manual of emotional intelligence scale.* National Psychological Corporation Agra.

Janoušková, M., Weissová, A., Formánek, T., Pasz, J., & Bankovská Motlová, L. (2017). Mental illness stigma among medical students and teachers. *International Journal of Social Psychiatry, 63*(8), 744–751.

Jorm, A. F., & Wright, A. (2008). Influences on young people's stigmatising attitudes towards peers with mental disorders: National survey of young Australians and their parents. *The British Journal of Psychiatry, 192*(2), 144–149.

Kessler, R. C., Berglund, P. A., Bruce, M. L., Koch, J. R., Laska, E. M., Leaf, P. J., Manderscheid, R. W., Rosenheck, R. A., Walters, E. E., & Wang, P. S. (2001). The prevalence and correlates of untreated serious mental illness. *Health Services Research, 36*(6 Pt 1), 987.

Kim-Cohen, J., & Turkewitz, R. (2012). Resilience and measured gene–environment interactions. *Development and Psychopathology, 24*(4), 1297–1306.

Komiya, N., Good, G. E., & Sherrod, N. B. (2000). Emotional openness as a predictor of college students' attitudes toward seeking psychological help. *Journal of counseling psychology, 47*(1), 138.

Kondrat, D. C., Sullivan, W. P., Wilkins, B., Barrett, B. J., & Beerbower, E. (2018). The mediating effect of social support on the relationship between the impact of experienced stigma and mental health. *Stigma and Health, 3*(4), 305.

Levitt, M. J., Weber, R. A., & Guacci, N. (1993). Convoys of social support: An intergenerational analysis. *Psychology and Aging, 8*(3), 323.

Losada, A., Márquez-González, M., García-Ortiz, L., Gómez-Marcos, M. A., Fernández-Fernández, V., & Rodríguez-Sánchez, E. (2012). Loneliness and mental health in a representative sample of community-dwelling Spanish older adults. *The Journal of psychology, 146*(3), 277–292.

Miville, M. L., & Constantine, M. G. (2006). Sociocultural predictors of psychological help-seeking attitudes and behavior among Mexican American college students. *Cultural Diversity and Ethnic Minority Psychology, 12*(3), 420.

Mojtabai, R., Olfson, M., Sampson, N. A., Jin, R., Druss, B., Wang, P. S., ... & Kessler, R. C. (2011). Barriers to mental health treatment: results from the National Comorbidity Survey Replication. *Psychological medicine, 41*(8), 1751–1761.

Nishi, D., Matsuoka, Y., & Kim, Y. (2010). Posttraumatic growth, posttraumatic stress disorder and resilience of motor vehicle accident survivors. *Biopsychosocial medicine, 4*(1), 1–6.

Offer, D., Howard, K. I., Schonert, K. A., & Ostrov, E. (1991). To whom do adolescents turn for help? Differences between disturbed and nondisturbed adolescents. *Journal of the American Academy of Child & Adolescent Psychiatry, 30*(4), 623–630.

Parker, R. G., & Parrott, R. (1995). Patterns of self-disclosure across social support networks: Elderly, middle-aged, and young adults. *The International Journal of Aging and Human Development, 41*(4), 281–297.

Parslow, R. A., & Jorm, A. F. (2000). Who uses mental health services in Australia? An analysis of data from the national survey of mental health and wellbeing. *Australian & New Zealand Journal of Psychiatry, 34*(6), 997–1008.

Pierce, M., Hope, H., Ford, T., Hatch, S., Hotopf, M., John, A., Kontopantelis, E., Webb, R., Wessely, S., Mcmanus, S., & Abel, K. M. (2020). Mental health before and during the COVID-19 pandemic: A longitudinal probability sample survey of the UK population. *The Lancet Psychiatry, 7*(10), 883–892.

Rickwood, D. J., & Braithwaite, V. A. (1994). Social-psychological factors affecting help-seeking for emotional problems. *Social Science & Medicine, 39*(4), 563–572.

Rickwood, D., Deane, F. P., Wilson, C. J., & Ciarrochi, J. (2005). Young people's help-seeking for mental health problems. *Australian e-journal for the Advancement of Mental health, 4*(3), 218–251.

Seidman, A. J., Crick, K. A., & Wade, N. G. (2022). Personal growth initiative, mental health stigma, and intentions to seek professional psychological help: A model extension. *Stigma and Health, 7*(2), 142–151.

Wagnild, G. (2009). A review of the resilience scale. *Journal of Nursing Measurement, 17*(2), 105–113.

Wagnild, G. M., & Young, H. M. (1993). Development and psychometric. *Journal of nursing measurement, 1*(2), 165–178.

Wolska, A., & Pietrulewicz, B. (2008). Attitudes toward people with mental illness (stigma) in the intercultural context. *Polish Journal of Social Science, 3*, 213–240.

Zimet, G. D., Dahlem, N. W., Zimet, S. G., & Farley, G. K. (1988). The multidimensional scale of perceived social support. *Journal of personality assessment, 52*(1), 30–41.

3 Quality of Living in the Aftermath of a Pandemic

Sukanya Chowdhury, Turfa Ahmed and Tilottama Mukherjee

Introduction

The decade ushered in a novel virus that brought the world to a complete standstill overnight. Countries sealed their gates, and citizens were advised to stay under lockdown for as long as the situation demanded. Soon after it surfaced, the severe acute respiratory syndrome (SARS-CoV-2) COVID-19 virus resulted in an outbreak that raised grave public health concerns across the globe. The World Health Organization (WHO) declared it a global pandemic by March 2020, taking note of the global spread of the disease affecting citizens of several countries. The primary focus was to prevent the wide-scale spread of a disease that had severe medical ramifications. However, endangered physical health is not the only consequence of a pandemic. A pandemic leaves an equally devastating impact on the Mental Health of individuals. It has a host of subtle and far-reaching effects on our psyche that individuals often ignore. The consequences are borne by societies for years to come, often leading to anxiety, PTSD, severe depression, or burnout.

Governments in various countries adopted strict lockdown and quarantine measures to deal with the crisis at hand. People were advised to follow social distancing protocols, always wear a mask when stepping outside their homes, wash their hands, and sanitise their surroundings constantly. The closure of public places such as offices, educational institutes, and entertainment venues confined people to their homes (Javed et al., 2020). A global health phenomenon of this nature has significant repercussions on our well-being and quality of life. Psychological distress in the general population is a common by-product of any pandemic that often manifests itself in the form of related symptoms such as panic, anxiety, and sadness, to name a few (Wang et al., 2019). The restrictive measures have gravely affected the social and Mental Health of individuals across the world. A review published in *The Lancet* reported that the separation from loved ones, loss of freedom, boredom, and uncertainty could cause a deterioration in an individual's Mental

DOI: 10.4324/9781003348429-3

Health status (Yao et al., 2020). Literature shows that factors like extended periods of quarantine, loneliness, confinement, fear of contracting the virus, concerns regarding the health of family members, loss of jobs, financial difficulties, and inadequate information can play a role in facilitating poor Mental Health and worsening our quality of life (Serafini et al., 2020).

The World Health Organization describes Quality of Life as an individual's perception of their standing in life about the society they are living in and concerning their goals and standards. It is a subjective measure of an individual's happiness and degree of satisfaction with their day-to-day living. Factors such as financial security, job satisfaction, family life, health, and safety play an important role in determining our quality of life. In recent times, many individuals have undergone *"massive changes in their lives, involving their health, employment, and family life"* (Xiao et al., 2020; Gangopadhyaya & Garrett, 2020). Such an accumulation of multiple stressors elevates the chances of developing psychological distress and a decreased sense of well-being. It would be reasonable to assume that a crisis of this magnitude that gave rise to uncertainty and fear among the masses would witness a change in the quality of living. How we adjust to adverse life situations alters the quality of our lives. These circumstances bring their share of positive and negative life changes. How we adjust to such changes is also influenced by several factors such as our personality, attitude to life, cognitive functioning, and resilience in the face of challenges. Mental Health professionals argue that resilient individuals can effectively adapt to dynamic situations during a crisis, reducing their vulnerability to adverse outcomes (Haldane et al., 2021). Literature from previous epidemics, such as Ebola and severe acute respiratory syndrome (SARS), displays the connection between resilience and thwarting new outbreak transmission (Nuzzo et al., 2019). The American Psychological Association (APA, 2020) describes resilience as "how people adapt well to adversities, trauma, life-threatening tragedies, or other signs such stressors-like any physical, psychological, financial or environmental stressors." Not only does resilience involve "bouncing back" from such strenuous experiences, but the resultant profound personal growth helps the individual to overcome challenges and grow through difficult phases of life as well.

The authors thus hypothesised that resilience would play an important role in cushioning the impact of the pandemic, which in turn would influence the quality of life of a population that faced one of the worst crises in the history of humankind.

Method

The present study explored the impact of COVID-19 on general health, quality of life, and resilience among adults, essentially COVID-19 survivors in India.

We conducted a cross-sectional study from March 2021 to August 2021 in Kolkata, India. The data was collected through the snowball sampling method. Participants' consent was taken before they filled up the questionnaires. The participants were presented with five questionnaires which were an Information Schedule, the Impact of Event Scale – Revised (IES-R; Weiss & Marmar, 1997), the World Health Organization Quality of Life – B.R.E.F. (WHOQOL-BREF; WHOQOL Group, 1998), the General Health Questionnaire-12 (GHQ-12; Goldberg & Williams, 1988), and the abbreviated version of Nicholson McBride Resilience Questionnaire (N.M.R.Q.; Clarke & Nicholson, 2010).

The IES-R asked the respondents to rate the difficulties or distress they faced after stressful life events, particularly concerning COVID-19, on a five-point Likert scale ranging from "Not at all" to "Extremely." The WHO-QOL-BREF asked the respondents to rate their feelings about their quality of life, health or other areas of life, standards, hopes, pleasures, and concerns in the past two weeks on a five-point Likert scale ranging from "Not at all/Never/ Very dissatisfied/Very poor" to "Completely/ Always/ Very satisfied/Extremely." The GHQ-12 was used as a tool, consisting of six positively and six negatively worded items, to assess the severity of psychological morbidity (such as anxiety, depression, or social dysfunction) on a four-point Likert scale ranging from "much less than usual" to "more so than usual" in case of positive statements and "not at all" to "much more than usual" in case of negative statements. The responses were scored using the Likert method, and a higher score on GHQ-12 indicated worse Mental Health than those scoring lower on the scale. The NMRQ required the respondents to rate their answers on a Likert scale of five points ranging from "Strongly agree" on one end to "Strongly disagree" on the other.

The total sample (N = 120) was divided into two groups, one group consisted of the COVID-19 survivors (n = 60), and the other group consisted of individuals who had not contracted COVID-19 (n = 60). Participants in the COVID-19 group were selected keeping in mind the following inclusion criteria. The participants had to be aged between 20 and 50 years with a confirmed diagnosis of COVID-19 in the past year. In the case of the non-COVID-19 group, participants between the ages of 20 and 50 years without any medical history of COVID-19 symptoms were selected. Individuals who displayed symptoms of COVID-19 in the past year but had not received a clinical diagnosis of the same were excluded from the present study.

Based on the obtained data, statistical analysis was conducted using the Statistical Package for Social Sciences (SPSS), Windows Version 16.0.

Results

Table 3.1 summarises the mean and standard deviations of all the variables considered in the present study: the impact of event, general health, quality

Table 3.1 Descriptive statistics for the COVID-19 and non-COVID-19 groups

	COVID-19 (N = 60)		Non-COVID-19 (N = 60)	
	Mean	Std. Deviation	Mean	Std. Deviation
GHQ-12	13.2308	6.41571	16.1579	7.27714
Impact of Event				
Intrusion	.8212	.78672	1.4959	.99665
Avoidance	.8061	.84290	1.5768	1.39249
Hyperarousal	.9951	1.22875	1.4834	1.07434
Total	18.1154	17.46105	32.4211	20.96506
Quality of Life				
Physical	14.2500	2.51953	13.0877	2.56543
Psychological	13.3269	2.48699	12.1404	2.74798
Social	14.3462	3.12413	13.3684	3.00970
Environment	14.6538	2.23944	13.5965	2.56946
Resilience	43.8269	7.17217	41.8947	7.55618

Source: Author/s

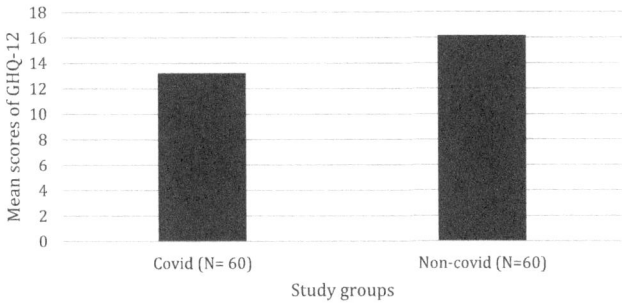

Figure 3.1 Comparison of the GHQ-12 Scores Between the COVID-19 and Non-COVID-19 Group

Source: Author/s

of life, and resilience. The comparative representation of the mean scores has been shown in Figures 3.1, 3.2, 3.3, and 3.4, respectively.

Tables 3.2 and 3.3 represent the correlation between the various variables considered in the present study. The present study found a significant association of general health with the impact of event and quality of life in the COVID-19 survivors. Additionally, the impact of event is significantly associated with quality of life, and resilience is significantly associated with the psychological aspect of quality of life among COVID-19 survivors. Whereas, among the individuals who did not contract the COVID-19 virus, general health is significantly associated with the impact of event, quality

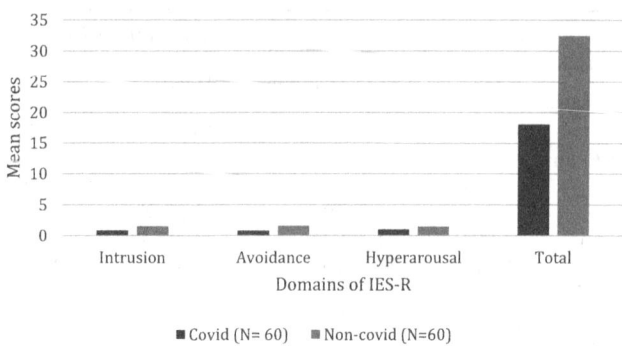

Figure 3.2 Comparison of the Impact of Event Scale – Revised (IES-R) Scores Between the COVID-19 and Non-COVID-19 Group

Source: Author/s

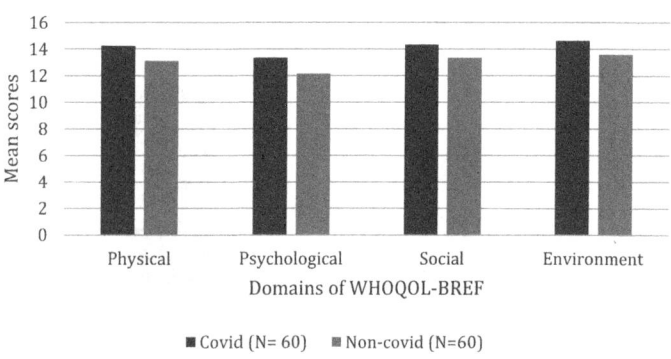

Figure 3.3 Comparison of the World Health Organization Quality of Life Scale (WHOQOL-BREF) Scores Between the COVID-19 and Non-COVID-19 Group

Source: Author/s

of life, and resilience. The impact of event has also been found to be significantly associated with quality of life and resilience. The quality of life has also been found to be significantly associated with resilience among this group.

Table 3.4 represents the significant differences between the scores of both groups for all the variables considered in the present study.

Table 3.5 summarises the causal factors for the variables considered in the present study. The table shows that hyperarousal caused by an impactful event is a predictor of resilience in the present study. The overall impact of

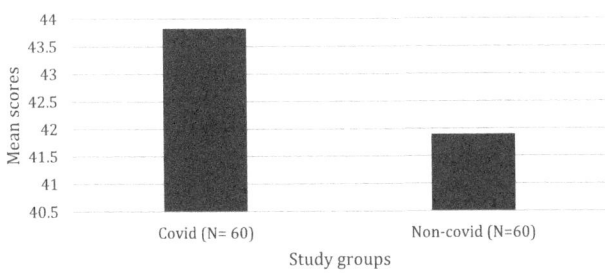

Figure 3.4 Comparison of the Resilience Scores Between the COVID-19 and Non-COVID-19 Group

Source: Author/s

an event significantly influences the physical, psychological, and environmental aspects of quality of life. Resilience is a consistent predictor of all aspects of quality of life in the present study. The intrusion caused by an impactful event significantly affects the social aspect of quality of life as well. The physical and psychological quality of life predicts the experience of the general health of individuals in the present study.

Discussion

In the past 2 years, during humankind's struggle with COVID-19, there have been profound changes in our perception of the world around us. New ways of living have been introduced, and our day-to-day interactions and activities have undergone significant alterations. Changes like these leave their imprints on the human mind, thus, in turn affecting our attitude towards life, behaviour, and general quality of living. Findings from a recent study reported that the disruption caused due to the pandemic in people's work, family, or social life had unique contributions to poor Mental Health (Hansel et al., 2022). The results of the current work revealed quite a few interesting findings for the variables studied among COVID-19 survivors and their non-affected counterparts.

The findings reveal significant differences between both groups in the General Health Questionnaire (GHQ-12), with COVID-19 survivors reporting a lower mean score, thus indicating a better condition of their current Mental Health status than the non-affected individuals. This finding is consistent with Dienstbier's argument that limited exposure to stressors along with an opportunity for recovery has a positive toughening effect on individuals (Seery, 2010). The current study involves survivors of COVID-19 who returned to normal functioning in their daily lives after their period of quarantine and recovery. Most of these individuals received proper

Table 3.2 Pearson's product moment correlation for COVID-19 group

	GHQ-12	IES_Intrusion	IES_Avoidance	IES_Hyperarousal	IES_Total	QOL_1	QOL_2	QOL_3	QOL_4	Resilience
GHQ-12	1	.695**	.577**	.599**	.719**	-.633**	-.636**	-.339*	-.327*	-.245
IES_Intrusion		1	.848**	.633**	.949**	-.468**	-.605**	-.483**	-.370**	-.227
IES_Avoidance			1	.599**	.937**	-.367**	-.468**	-.485**	-.259	-.188
IES_Hyperarousal				1	.700**	-.246	-.513**	-.453**	-.172	-.230
IES_Total					1	-.466**	-.603**	-.494**	-.356**	-.243
QOL_1						1	.625**	.367**	.599**	.203
QOL_2							1	.624**	.619**	.380**
QOL_3								1	.401**	.245
QOL_4									1	.221
Resilience										1

** Correlation is significant at the 0.01 level (p < 0.01). * Correlation is significant at the 0.05 level (p < 0.05).
GHQ-12 = General Health Questionnaire-12; IES= Impact of Event-Revised; QOL= Quality of Life; QOL_1= Quality of Life (Physical domain); QOL_2= Quality of Life (Psychological domain); QOL_3= Quality of Life (Social domain); QOL_4= Quality of Life (Environmental domain)

Source: Author/s

Table 3.3 Pearson's product moment correlation for non-COVID-19 group

	GHQ-12	IES_Intrusion	IES_Avoidance	IES_Hyperarousal	IES_Total	QOL_1	QOL_2	QOL_3	QOL_4	Resilience
GHQ-12	1	.527**	.264*	.570**	.519**	-.510**	-.430**	-.064	-.396**	-.462**
IES_Intrusion		1	.731**	.902**	.953**	-.591**	-.477**	-.422**	-.408**	-.262*
IES_Avoidance			1	.644**	.791**	-.407**	-.355**	-.348**	-.264*	-.282*
IES_Hyperarousal				1	.928**	-.720**	-.545**	-.358**	-.477**	-.356**
IES_Total					1	-.605**	-.485**	-.393**	-.419**	—.280*
QOL_1						1	.662**	.174	.420**	.398**
QOL_2							1	.413**	.572**	.531**
QOL_3								1	.431**	.227
QOL_4									1	.394**
Resilience										1

** Correlation is significant at the 0.01 level ($p < 0.01$). * Correlation is significant at the 0.05 level ($p < 0.05$).
GHQ-12 = General Health Questionnaire-12; IES = Impact of Event-Revised; QOL= Quality of Life, QOL_1 = Quality of Life (physical domain); QOL_2 = Quality of Life (psychological domain); QOL_3 = Quality of Life (social domain); QOL_4 = Quality of Life (environmental domain)

Source: Author/s

Table 3.4 Comparison between the COVID-19 and non-COVID-19 groups

Variables	$t_{(118)}$
GHQ-12	2.219*
Impact of Event	
Intrusion	3.898**
Avoidance	3.455**
Hyperarousal	2.213*
Total	3.850**
Quality of Life	
Physical	−2.383*
Psychological	−2.356*
Social	−1.664
Environment	−2.280*
Resilience	−1.366

*p < 0.05 – statistically significant; **p < 0.01 – statistically significant; GHQ-12 = General Health Questionnaire-12.

Source: Author/s

Table 3.5 Stepwise linear regression analysis

Criterion	Predictors	F Ratios	R	R^2	β	t Values
Resilience	IES_Hyperarousal	$F_{(1, 118)}= 11.432$**	.311	.097	−.311	−3.381**
QOL_1	Resilience	$F_{(1, 118)}= 12.827$**	.327	.107	.327	3.581**
	IES_Total	$F_{(1, 118)}= 52.886$**	.575	.331	−.575	−7.272**
QOL_2	Resilience	$F_{(1, 118)}= 31.769$**	.478	.229	.478	5.636**
	IES_Total	$F_{(1, 118)}= 49.865$**	.564	.318	−.564	−7.062**
QOL_3	Resilience	$F_{(1, 118)}= 7.206$**	.251	.063	.251	2.684**
	IES_Intrusion	$F_{(1, 118)}= 29.702$**	.466	.217	−.466	−5.450**
QOL_4	Resilience	$F_{(1, 118)}= 13.747$**	.337	.114	.337	3.708**
	IES_Total	$F_{(1, 118)}= 25.083$**	.436	.190	−.436	−5.008**
GHQ-12	QOL_1	$F_{(2, 117)}= 32.787$**	.618	.382	−.404	−3.962**
	QOL_2				−.272	−2.665**

*p < 0.05 – statistically significant; **p < 0.01 – statistically significant; GHQ-12 = General Health Questionnaire-12; IES = Impact of Event-Revised; QOL= Quality of Life, QOL_1= Quality of Life (physical domain); QOL_2 = Quality of Life (psychological domain); QOL_3 = Quality of Life (social domain); QOL_4 = Quality of Life (environmental domain).

Source: Author/s

treatment and care post their diagnosis; thus, when diagnosed with COVID-19, they had an opportunity to recover and heal. Dienstbier (1989, 1992) further argued that sheltering an individual from all stressors in life leads to a lack of toughness. Although sheltering from stressors may temporarily protect a person from distress, it would not reap long-term benefits in life. Sheltering does not allow skills like toughness and mastery to develop, and neither does it persist indefinitely, so when stressors are eventually encountered, individuals are likely to be ill-equipped to cope with them. Coping with some amount of stress could help promote our perceptions of control and mastery over adverse situations in life. Thus, when survivors of COVID-19 were exposed to this life-threatening virus but made a complete recovery, it could instil in them a sense of mastery and a more remarkable ability to cope with life's adversities. On the other hand, individuals not affected by COVID-19 even though they were immune to the virus could be more apprehensive of its effects, worsening their Mental Health.

A significant positive association was found between GHQ-12 and all the Impact of Event Scale – Revised (IES-R) subscales (Intrusion, Avoidance, Hyperarousal) in both the COVID-19 and non-COVID-19 group of respondents, thus indicating that the more significant the impact of the pandemic, the more severe is its effect on the Mental Health of both COVID-19 survivors and their non-affected counterparts. Similar findings have been reported by Al Dhaheri and colleagues in a study conducted among the inhabitants of the MENA (the Middle East and North Africa) region, where approximately 40% of the respondents had IES-R scores that indicated "moderate to severe disturbance" due to the pandemic (Al Dhaheri et al., 2021). The current study also revealed a significant negative correlation between GHQ-12 and all subscales of the Quality of Life questionnaire (Physical, Psychological, Social, Environmental) among COVID-19 survivors and a significant negative correlation between GHQ-12 and the Physical, Psychological, and Environmental domains among the non-COVID-19 participants. Existing literature shows the correlation between mental disorders like anxiety and depression and almost all domains of the Quality of Life Scale (Nouri et al., 2021). The present findings indicate that Mental Health deterioration is associated with a diminished quality of life on all fronts. The pandemic has severely affected the Mental Health of individuals across the globe: constant wearing of face masks, frequent handwashing, disinfecting surfaces, social distancing and quarantine of infected individuals, and fear of contracting the virus are constant stressors that have influenced daily life activities (Lee & You, 2020). Unemployment, reduced salaries, and economic difficulties increase an individual's vulnerability, leading to a lower quality of life (Algahtani et al., 2021).

The present study also revealed a significant negative association between general health and resilience among participants in the non-COVID-19 group compared to the COVID-19 group. The findings can be strengthened by previous studies that have found a negative relationship between anxiety and individual resilience. It may be assumed that such individuals might have experienced a higher sense of danger due to the pandemic that might have enhanced their anxiety and apprehension levels, but a stronger sense of resilience may have declined this trend (Zizolfi et al., 2019; Kimhi et al., 2020). The higher GHQ-12 scores in the non-COVID-19 group could also be attributed to previous studies conducted during disease outbreaks. The fear of oneself or significant others contracting the disease might provoke anxiety and thus negatively influences both physical and psychological outcomes (Reynolds et al., 2008; Brooks et al., 2020), thereby, affecting the well-being of the individuals as well (Coulombe et al., 2020). Previous studies also corroborate the present findings that resilience is one of the most substantial contributors to Mental Health (Ellen et al., 2021) during a pandemic because of the need to cope with the stressors and attempt to minimise mental distress (Chen & Bonanno, 2020), as indicated by higher GHQ-12 scores and the subsequent lower scores on resilience and quality of life in the non-COVID-19 group.

Such an adverse and stressful event is influenced by protective factors such as resilience (Southwick et al., 2014). In the case of the present study, the IES-R scores were found to be significantly higher in the non-COVID-19 group and were found to have a significant negative association with resilience in the non-COVID-19 group but not in the COVID-19 group. A significant negative association was found between resilience and IES-R subscales, namely, Intrusion, Avoidance, and Hyperarousal in the non-COVID-19 group but not in the COVID-19 group in the present study. A study (Roy et al., 2020) reported that greater than 80% of the individuals were preoccupied with thoughts about the pandemic. Hyperarousal was found to predict resilience in the present study negatively. Bala et al. (2020) reported in their study that individuals scored high on the chances of developing preoccupation with intrusive thoughts related to the pandemic, the subsequent apprehension thus leading to hyperarousal symptoms and avoidance behaviour among them. Such ruminative thoughts may have affected individuals' Mental Health during the pandemic by practising behaviours to avoid the risk of being sick such as (but not limited to) gaining more information from sources at their disposal or by following adequate safety protocols and avoiding distressing feelings, ideas, or situations related to the pandemic or numbing of responsiveness. Therefore, in a bid to escape the pandemic through survival strategies, the Mental Health indexes in the non-COVID-19 group might have become lower compared to those who contracted COVID-19 virus. Thus, this might have affected the resilience scores significantly in the non-COVID-19 group. It might be suggested that individuals who have already dealt with the sickness had to resign to the circumstances and endure an arduous recovery process. So, they might have been better able to adapt to the novel and evolving situation during the pandemic because of their prior experience with isolation and a loss of activity due to their ill health, and it, therefore, prepared them to cope better with the present crisis. Recent studies have reported that individuals developed more resistance to the pandemic and the corresponding restrictions over time, perhaps because of being accustomed to the frequent changes in policies that further enhanced their adaptation to uncertainty. Their coping with the events related to the pandemic enhanced their adjustment to changes in daily life, thereby reducing the impact of the pandemic on the quality of life overtime (Mohsen et al., 2022; Brinkhof et al., 2021; Hussong et al., 2022). However, the higher IES-R scores among the individuals in the non-COVID-19 group increase their risk of developing stress-related psychopathologies later, as reported by previous studies (Ifthikar et al., 2021; Sood, 2020).

The current findings reveal significant differences between both groups in three dimensions of the WHO-QoL questionnaire, namely the physical, psychological, and environmental dimensions, with the COVID-19 group reporting higher mean scores, which indicates a better quality of life. The present findings can be explained in light of the Post Traumatic Growth (PTG) Theory. Developed by psychologists Richard Tedeschi and Lawrence Calhoun in the mid-1990s, PTG is the idea that, in the long run, traumatic events and experiences – like illness, accidents, bereavement – can have beneficial effects. Often when individuals come face to face with a traumatic situation in their lives, after recovering from the initial shock stage, people report feeling more appreciative of their lives (Tedeschi & Calhoun, 1996). They discover new inner strength. They feel self-assured in the face of life's challenges. They feel that their relationships are more intimate and authentic, and there is a newfound meaning and purpose in their lives. Survivors of COVID-19 have already faced and recovered from the worst; hence, it can be presumed considering current findings that there has been some growth, a newfound appreciation for life, leading them to have a better quality of life than the non-COVID-19 group of individuals who are living in a constant fear of contracting the illness every day.

For the present sample, all dimensions of Quality of Life have been found to have a significant negative association with the total Impact of Event scale scores among both groups of participants, thus indicating that the impact the pandemic has had on people's lives, such as quarantining, living in isolation, separation from loved ones, financial loss, adoption of constant precautionary measures, has greatly diminished all aspects of our quality of life. For the non-COVID-19 group of participants, the physical, psychological, and environmental dimensions of quality of life have positive associations with resilience, and in the case of COVID-19 survivors, the psychological dimension of Quality of Life was positively associated with resilience, thus highlighting the importance of resilience in maintaining our psychological well-being. Resilience allows individuals to maintain a healthy outcome even amidst adverse situations and rebound after facing setbacks in life (Rutter, 2007; Silver, 2009).

In the present study, the higher mean score on the psychological dimension of the WHO-QoL scale for the COVID-19 group could be attributed to the process of PTG. Similar findings have been reported in a study by Li and Hu (2022), where PTG was found to have a positive association with Psychological Resilience, with factors such as positive coping styles and cognitive reappraisal mediating the association between the two. A process such as PTG influences our overall psychological well-being, and looking back at adverse situations as opportunities to learn and grow from allows people to be more appreciative of their lives. It instils a sense of self assurance and confidence to be able to handle life's challenges in a more effective manner.

In the current study, the physical and psychological dimensions of quality of life are also predictors of general health, thus indicating that a good quality of life, especially related to individuals' physical and psychological health, dramatically affects our general health and psychological well-being. Mental and physical well-being are two sides of the same coin, interwoven faculties that govern a person's overall health. The pandemic and the lockdown measures have significantly impacted people's lives, causing excessive anxiety, distress and panic, depression, and post-traumatic symptoms (Holmes et al., 2020; Brooks et al., 2020). Hence, a diminished physical and psychological quality of life could not guarantee an individual's good health and well-being on either front.

Limitations of the current study and future directions

If the sample size of the study were larger, it could have increased the generalisability of the findings in the population. Future research conducted with a larger sample size could lead to further findings. Additionally, all the measures were self-report rating scales in this study. In future research, this could be supplemented with information gathered from the sample with qualitative semi-structured interviews by trained examiners. Since the data gathered for this research process was web-based, there is a possibility that it might have led to a selection bias towards only those privileged with literacy and access to technological resources.

The study's findings suggest that survivors of COVID-19 overall had a better Mental Health index in terms of their general health and quality of life, whereas the overall impact of this event was more severe for the group of participants not diagnosed with COVID-19. In addition, resilience had a significant negative association with general health for this group of participants. In the current study, resilience is also a significant predictor for all domains of Quality of Life and general health. The constant apprehension to evade the disease and lower resistance in the face of adversity might have impacted their overall quality of life, which is significantly lower than that of the survivors of COVID-19. Hence, this affirms the finding that a lower degree of resilience can lead to poor quality of life. The inability to cope with the impact of a traumatic situation can have lasting effects on our general health and psychological well-being.

References

Al Dhaheri, A. S., Bataineh, M. F., Mohamad, M. N., Ajab, A., Al Marzouqi, A., Jarrar, A. H., Habib-Mourad, C., Abu Jamous, D. O., Ali, H. I., Al Sabbah, H., & Hasan, H. (2021). Impact of COVID-19 on mental health and quality of life: Is there any effect? A cross-sectional study of the MENA region. *PLoS One*, *16*(3), e0249107.

Algahtani, F. D., Hassan, S. N., Alsaif, B., & Zrieq, R. (2021). Assessment of the quality of life during COVID-19 pandemic: A cross-sectional survey from the Kingdom of Saudi Arabia. *International Journal of Environmental Research and Public Health*, *18*(3), 847.

American Psychological Association. (2020). *Building your resilience*. www.apa. org/topics/resilience

Bala, S., Pandve, H., Manna, R., Sreelal, B. S., Patel, S., Saxena, T., & Joy, S. G. (2020). Impact of COVID-19 pandemic on mental health among Indians: A post-traumatic stress disorder. *Industrial Psychiatry Journal*, *29*, 251–256.

Brinkhof, L. P., Huth, K. B. S., Murre, J. M. J., de Wit, S., Krugers, H. J., Ridderink-hof, K. R. (2021). The interplay between quality of life and resilience factors in later life: A network analysis. *Frontiers in Psychology*, *12*, 752564.

Brooks, S. K., Webster, R. K., Smith, L. E., Woodland, L., Wessely, S., Greenberg, N., & Rubin, G. J. (2020). The psychological impact of quarantine and how to reduce it: A rapid review of the evidence. *The Lancet*, *395*(10227), 912–920.

Chen, S., & Bonanno, G. A. (2020). Psychological adjustment during the global outbreak of COVID-19: A resilience perspective. *Psychological Trauma: Theory, Research, Practice, and Policy*, *12*(S1), S51–S54.

Clarke, J., & Nicholson, J. (2010). *Resilience: Bounce back from whatever life throws at you*. Hachette.

Coulombe, S., Pacheco, T., Cox, E., Khalil, C., Doucerain, M. M., Auger, E., & Meunier, S. (2020). Risk and resilience factors during the COVID-19 pandemic: A snapshot of the experiences of Canadian workers early on in the crisis. *Frontiers in Psychology*, *11*, 580702.

Dienstbier, R. A. (1989). Arousal and physiological toughness: Implications for mental and physical health. *Psychological Review*, *96*, 84–100.

Dienstbier, R. A. (1992). Mutual impacts of toughening on crises and losses. In L. Montada, S. H. Filipp, & M. J. Lerner (Eds.), *Life crises and experiences of loss in adulthood* (pp. 367–384). Erlbaum.

Ellen, C., Patricia, D. V., Miet, D. L., Peter, V., Patrick, C., Robby, D. P., Kristine, O., Maria, R. B., Arnaud, S., Antonio, M. B. J., Judit, F. S. A., Laura, V. M., & de Velde Dominique, V. (2021). Meaningful activities during COVID-19 lockdown and association with mental health in Belgian adults. *B.M.C. Public Health*, *21*(1).

Gangopadhyaya, A., & Garrett, A. B. (2020). Unemployment, health insurance, and the COVID-19 recession. *SSRN Journal*, 1–8.

Goldberg, D. P., & Williams, P. (1988). *A user's guide to the general health questionnaire.* NFER-Nelson.

Haldane, V., De Foo, C., Abdalla, S. M., Jung, A. S., Tan, M., Wu, S., Chua, A., Verma, M., Shrestha, P., Singh, S., & Perez, T. (2021). Health systems resilience in managing the COVID-19 pandemic: Lessons from 28 countries. *Nature Medicine, 27*, 964–980.

Hansel, T. C., Saltzman, L. Y., Melton, P. A., Clark, T. L., & Bordnick, P. S. (2022). COVID-19 behavioral health and quality of life. *Scientific Reports, 12*, 961.

Holmes, E. A., O'Connor, R. C., Perry, V. H., Tracey, I., Wessely, S., Arseneault, L., Ballard, C. G., Christensen, H., Cohen Silver, R., Everall, I., Ford, T., John, A., Kabir, T., King, K., Madan, I., Michie, S., Przybylski, A. K., Shafran, R., Sweeney, A., . . . Bullmore, E. (2020). Multidisciplinary research priorities for the COVID-19 pandemic: A call for action for mental health science. *Lancet Psychiatry, 7*(6), 547–560.

Hussong, J., Moehler, E., Kühn, A., Wenning, M., Gehrke, T., Burckhart, H., Richter, U., Nonnenmacher, A., Zemlin, M., Lücke, T., & Brinkmann, F. (2022). Mental health and health-related quality of life in German adolescents after the third wave of the COVID-19 pandemic. *Children, 9*(6).

Ifthikar, Z., Fakih, S. S., Johnson, S., & Alex, J. (2021). Post-traumatic stress disorder following COVID-19 pandemic among medical students in Riyadh: A cross-sectional study. *Middle East Current Psychiatry, 28*, 44.

Javed, B., Sarwer, A., Soto, E. B., & Mashwani, Z. R. (2020). Is Pakistan's response to coronavirus (SARS-CoV-2) adequate to prevent an outbreak? *Frontiers in Medicine, 7*, 1–4.

Kimhi, S., Eshel, Y., Marciano, H., & Adini, B. (2020). Distress and resilience in the days of COVID-19: Comparing two ethnicities. *International Journal of Environmental Research and Public Health, 17*(11), 3956.

Lee, M., & You, M. (2020). Psychological and behavioral responses in South Korea during the early stages of coronavirus disease 2019 (COVID-19). *International Journal of Environmental Research and Public Health, 17*, 2977.

Li, Q., & Hu, J. (2022). Post traumatic growth and psychological resilience during the COVID-19 pandemic: A serial mediation model. *Frontiers in Psychiatry, 13*, 1–11.

Mohsen, S., El-Masry, R., Ali, O. F., & Abdel-Hady, D. (2022). Quality of life during COVID-19 pandemic: A community-based study in Dakahlia governorate, Egypt. *Global Health Research and Policy, 7*, 15.

Nouri, F., Feizi, A., Roohafza, H., Sadeghi, M., & Sarrafzadegan, N. (2021). How different domains of quality of life are associated with latent dimensions of mental health measured by GHQ-12. *Health and Quality of Life Outcomes, 19*, 255.

Nuzzo, B., Meyer, D., Snyder, M., Ravi, S. J., Lapascu, A., Souleles, J., Andrada, C. I., & Bishai, D. (2019). What makes health systems resilient against infectious disease outbreaks and natural hazards? Results from a scoping review. *BMC Public Health, 19*, 1310.

Reynolds, D. L., Garay, J. R., Deamond, S. L., Moran, M. K., Gold, W., & Styra, R. (2008). Understanding, compliance and psychological impact of the SARS quarantine experience. *Epidemiology and Infection, 136*, 997–1007.

Roy, D., Tripathy, S., Kar, S. K., Sharma, N., Verma, S. K., & Kaushalb, V. (2020). Study of knowledge, attitude, anxiety and perceived mental healthcare needs in Indian population during COVID-19 pandemic. *Asian Journal of Psychiatry*, *51*, 102083.

Rutter, M. (2007). Resilience, competence, and coping. *Child Abuse and Neglect*, *31*, 205–209.

Seery, M. D., Holman, E. A., & Silver, R. C. (2010). Whatever does not kill us: Cumulative lifetime adversity, vulnerability, and resilience. *Journal of Personality and Social Psychology*, *99*(6), 1025–1041.

Serafini, G., Parmigiani, B., Amerio, A., Aguglia, A., Sher, L., & Amore, M. (2020). The psychological impact of COVID-19 on mental health in the general population. *QJM: An International Journal of Medicine*, *113*(8), 531–537.

Silver, R. C. (2009). Resilience. In D. Sander & K. Scherer (Eds.), *The Oxford companion to emotion and the affective sciences* (p. 343). Oxford University Press.

Sood, S. (2020). Psychological effects of the coronavirus disease-2019 pandemic. *Research & Humanities in Medical Education*, *7*, 23–26.

Southwick, S. M., Bonanno, G. A., Masten, A. S., Panter-Brick, C., & Yehuda, R. (2014). Resilience definitions, theory, and challenges: Interdisciplinary perspectives. *European Journal of Psychotraumatology*, *5*, 25338.

Tedeschi, R. G., & Calhoun, L. G. (1996). The post traumatic growth inventory: Measuring the positive legacy of trauma. *The Journal of Traumatic Stress*, *9*(3), 455–471.

Wang, C., Pan, R., Wan, X., Tan, Y., Xu, L., Ho, C. S., & Ho., R. (2020). Immediate psychological responses and associated factors during the initial stage of the 2019 coronavirus disease (COVID-19) epidemic among the general population in China. *International Journal of Environmental Research and Public Health*, *17*(5), 1729.

Weiss, D. S., & Marmar, C. R. (1997). The impact of event scale – revised. In J. P. Wilson & T. M. Keane (Eds.), *Assessing psychological trauma and PTSD* (pp. 399–411). Guilford Press.

WHOQOL Group. (1998). Development of the world health organization WHOQOL-BREF quality of life assessment: The WHOQOL group. *Psychological Medicine*, *28*(3), 551–558.

Xiao, H., Zhang, Y., Kong, D., Li, S., & Yang, N. (2020). The effects of social support on sleep quality of medical staff treating patients with coronavirus disease 2019 (COVID-19) in January and February 2020 in China. *Medical Science Monitor*, *26*, e923549–e923541.

Yao, H., Chen, J. H., & Xu, Y. F. (2020). Patients with mental health disorders in the COVID-19 epidemic. *Lancet Psychiatry*, *7*(4), 21.

Zizolfi, D., Poloni, N., Caselli, I., Ielmini, M., Lucca, G., Diurni, M., Cavallini, G., & Callegari, C. (2019). Resilience and recovery style: A retrospective study on associations among personal resources, symptoms, neurocognition, quality of life and psychosocial functioning in psychotic patients. *Psychology Research and Behavior Management*, *12*, 385–395.

4 Impact of Loneliness and Cognitive Emotion Regulation in Psychological Well-being of Students During the Pandemic

Urmimala Ghose and Tilottama Mukherjee

Introduction

The COVID-19 epidemic, which began in 2020, drastically affected people's lives and perceptions of the world. The impacts of the infection itself, combined with the containment efforts, have resulted in greater social isolation, financial insecurity, and worry about the future (Van Bavel et al., 2020). Many nations used non-pharmacological interventions such as social distancing measures to prevent the spread of the virus, while they awaited the discovery of an effective vaccine (Ferguson et al., 2020). The pandemic and the social distancing methods adopted to contain it have had devastating Mental Health implications (Holmes et al., 2020). In this context, it is crucial to comprehend how the pandemic has affected psychological well-being, as well as how varied individual characteristics make individuals more mentally prone or robust to its adverse impacts (Van Bavel et al., 2020).

Consistent with the eudemonic perspective, Ryff (1989) defined psychological well-being as the degree to which individuals believe they have meaningful influence over their lives and activities and are specifically concerned with their growth and self-realization. She put forward a composite and multidimensional model that served as the foundation for this research. It comprises the following dimensions: comprising self-acceptance, positive relations with others, autonomy, environmental mastery, personal growth, and purpose in life. These dimensions focus on individuals' various capacities to regulate their behaviour, assume the demands of the context, develop individual potential through positive interpersonal relationships, accept their limitations while maintaining a positive attitude, and find meaning and direction in their own lives (Keyes, 2002).

Loneliness has also been defined from various perspectives by different researchers. Sociologist Robert S. Weiss defines loneliness as "a response to the absence of some particular type of relationship or, more accurately, a response to the absence of some particular relational provision" (1973,

DOI: 10.4324/9781003348429-4

p. 17), and the current study is based on this typology of loneliness. Weiss (1973) further categorized loneliness into emotional loneliness, resulting from lack of a close, intimate attachment to another person, and social loneliness, stemming from an impoverished social network.

Emotion regulation is defined as all of an individual's conscious and unconscious techniques for reducing, maintaining, or increasing pleasant or negative emotions (Gross, 2001). Within this framework, Garnefski and Kraaij (2007) describe cognitive emotion regulation as the conscious monitoring and manipulating information that leads to emotional arousal. There are nine cognitive strategies that can be classified into two major categories: adaptive cognitive coping (e.g. planning, positive reappraisal, positive refocusing, putting into perspective, and acceptance), which is linked to higher psychological adjustment and quality of life, and maladaptive cognitive coping (e.g. self-blame, blaming others, rumination, and catastrophizing), associated with psychological maladjustment and mental and physical health problems.

Planning refers to deciding on the steps to take towards finding a solution and appropriately handling an adverse event. Positive reappraisal refers to thoughts of giving the event a positive meaning in terms of personal growth. Positive refocusing emphasizes thinking about the good parts of one's experiences instead of focusing on the actual bad or stressful occurrence. Putting things into perspective is a method that involves attempting to minimize the significance of a dangerous or stressful occurrence. Acceptance is a strategy that involves accepting what has happened to oneself. Self-blaming is the act of blaming oneself for one's unpleasant experiences. Other-blame is the act of blaming others or the environment for one's poor experiences. Rumination happens when a person is concerned with or overthinks the sensations and ideas related to a negative incident. Catastrophizing refers to the idea of highlighting the unpleasant experiences a person has experienced.

Despite abundant evidence of the positive effects of social support on mental well-being as well as evidence of the link between loneliness and a variety of poor Mental Health outcomes, loneliness as a psychological factor has been studied in relation to psychological well-being components only rarely. Also, to date, most research has focused on the relationship between cognitive emotion regulation and distress symptoms to determine which techniques are risk (or protective) factors for emotional disorders and thus may be valuable targets for psychotherapy therapies (Garnefski & Kraaij, 2007). Surprisingly, few researches, on the other hand, have looked at whether the dispositional use of cognitive emotion regulation mechanisms in response to adversity is linked to positive elements of an individual's well-being, such as good psychological functioning and experience (Ben-Zur, 2009; Gross & John, 2003; Ryan & Deci, 2001).

This is a significant oversight since illness and well-being may be thought of as being largely separate realms of mental functioning, with knowledge of the correlates of one not necessarily extending to the other (Keyes, 2002; Ryan & Deci, 2001). To put it differently, well-being should be defined not just in terms of the absence of psychopathology but also in terms of human strengths and potentials (Seligman & Csikzentmihalyi, 2014).

Given the rising body of evidence demonstrating that young adults are more prone to loneliness (Luhman & Hawkley, 2016), it is crucial to explore the contribution of this factor to the well-being of students. Additionally, students are more likely to have adjustment issues, bodily difficulties, and psychological anguish (Constantine et al., 2004). This calls for applying strategies and resources to cope with these sources of stress to have both optimal levels of psychological well-being and continuation of their academic life satisfactorily. With the COVID-19 pandemic being a global crisis, students have been disproportionately impacted. In a recent Indian study, Gupta and Parimal (2020) pointed out that tensions connected to the quest for identity, worries for academic performance and career, and anxiety about the future have all intensified the difficulties faced by the students throughout this period.

Those having a tendency of employing maladaptive cognitive regulation strategies are more likely to have negative emotional symptoms. However, it has not been adequately considered which cognitive emotion regulation strategies are related to well-being in students during a health crisis, which is crucial for promoting the early identification of negative emotions and developing psychological interventions to enable them to participate in future events. As a result, this field of research is extremely promising and deserves more attention and interest, particularly given the limitations in social interactions consequent upon the pandemic. The current study, thus, seeks to determine how loneliness and the different cognitive emotion regulation strategies contribute to psychological well-being of young adults during the COVID-19 pandemic. It also examines whether cognitive emotion regulation explains well-being beyond loneliness.

Methods

Research Design

The first part of the study involved a *correlational design* in which we attempted to find out the relationship of the different components of loneliness and cognitive emotion regulation with those of psychological well-being of students during the COVID-19 pandemic. In the second part, which was *ex post facto*, attempts were made to find out the hierarchical contribution of different components of predictor variables, that is loneliness and cognitive emotion regulation, on predicting the components of the criterion variable, that is psychological well-being.

Participants

One hundred and eighteen students (mean age of 21.07 years, 67.8% female), recruited through purposive sampling, volunteered to participate in the study. The primary inclusion criteria were: age range 18–25 years, middle socioeconomic status, permanent residents of Kolkata and outskirts, minimum education level till higher secondary, can understand English, staying at their personal/rented residence since April 2020 till taking the survey and being enrolled in a regular degree course in online mode at least for the last 2 months, or have completed one in the last month. Respondents currently suffering from history of any self-declared pre-existing diagnosed psychological/chronic physical illness or that of any significant physical illness, including COVID-19 in the last month, were excluded from the study. The sociodemographic characteristics of the sample are described in Table 4.1.

Table 4.1 Sample description

	Frequency	*Percentage*
Total	118	100.00
Age group		
Below 21	54	45.76
21 and above	64	54.24
Sex		
Female	80	67.80
Male	38	32.20
Residential area		
Urban (Kolkata)	75	63.56
Semi-urban (outskirts)	43	36.44
Enrolment status in any regular academic course		
Currently enrolled	94	79.66
Not currently enrolled, but completed in the last month	24	20.34
Type of academic course		
Professional	62	52.54
Not-professional	56	47.46
Level of education		
Undergraduate	72	61.02
Postgraduate	46	38.98
Current status in a course		
Fresher	15	12.71

(Continued)

Table 4.1 (Continued)

	Frequency	Percentage
Intermediate	59	50.00
Outgoing	44	37.29
Relationship status		
Single	98	83.05
In a relationship	20	16.95
Household composition		
Living with family	118	100.00
Living alone	0	0.00
History of pre-existing diagnosed psychological/chronic physical illness		
Absent	118	100.00
Present	0	0.00
History of any significant physical illness other than SARS-CoV-2 in the last month		
Absent	118	100.00
Present	0	0.00
History of contracting SARS-CoV-2 since March 2020		
Absent	118	100.00
Present	0	0.00
Living condition since the outbreak of the pandemic		
A personal/rented residence	118	100.00
At shared residence (e.g. as paying guests, hostels)	0	0.00
History of self-quarantine due to SARS-CoV-2		
Present	48	40.68
Absent	70	59.32
Frequency of meeting a friend/relative in the last six months		
Haven't met one since lockdown	14	11.86
Less than once a month	50	42.37
Every month	20	16.95
Every week	16	13.56
Every few days	18	15.25
Most frequent means of communication with friends/ relatives in the last 6 months		
Phone calls	37	31.36
Video calls	31	26.27
Text messages	36	30.51
Other means of interactions	14	11.86

Source: Author/s

Materials

Information Schedule. The Information Schedule was used to know the basic sociodemographic details of the participants and certain information related to their general health and illness due to COVID-19.

Psychological Wellbeing Scale (Ryff, 1989). Psychological well-being was measured with Ryff's Psychological Wellbeing Scale (Ryff, 1989). The scale consisted of 42 items that are designed to measure six distinct dimensions of well-being, that is autonomy, environmental mastery, personal growth, positive relations with others, purpose in life, and self-acceptance, on a six-point Likert scale based on the respondents' degree of agreement to each statement, where 1 denotes "Strongly disagree" and 6 denotes "Strongly agree." A total is calculated for each subscale and for all the items to yield a global score. The higher score on every scale indicates that the respondent has more of that specific quality, and the sum of all scores indicates the overall psychological well-being. The reliabilities (Cronbach's alpha) ranged from 0.71 to 0.88 for Americans and 0.61 to 0.88 for Koreans, while those obtained in the present study ranged from 0.67 to 0.78 (refer to Table 4.2).

Loneliness Scale (de Jong-Gierveld & Kamphuls, 1985). To measure social and emotional loneliness, the De Jong Gierveld Loneliness Scale was used. It is an 11-item test developed in 1985, built on Weiss' research

Table 4.2 The means, standard deviations, and reliability coefficients of all variables for the total sample (N = 118)

Name of Variables With Components	Mean	Standard Deviation	Cronbach's α
Loneliness			
Emotional loneliness	2.06	0.98	0.78
Social loneliness	1.80	1.07	0.84
Cognitive emotion regulation			
Adaptive strategies			
Positive reappraisal	8.47	1.71	0.71
Planning	8.11	1.85	0.75
Acceptance	8.00	1.72	0.66
Putting into perspective	7.17	2.24	0.80
Positive refocusing	6.32	2.07	0.56
Maladaptive strategies			
Rumination	7.79	1.69	0.61
Self-blame	6.76	2.23	0.84
Catastrophizing	6.25	2.39	0.87
Other blame	4.80	1.80	0.81
Psychological well-being			
Personal growth	31.25	6.58	0.78
Positive relations	28.70	4.59	0.67
Purpose in life	27.43	4.98	0.69
Autonomy	27.03	6.43	0.72
Self-acceptance	25.49	7.63	0.84
Environmental mastery	25.32	4.81	0.68
Global psychological well-being	165.22	25.61	0.88

Source: Author/s

about loneliness as a concept of two components. It uses a five-point Likert scale ranging from 0 (none of the time) to 4 (all of the time). The scale has adequate internal consistency with a Cronbach's alpha of 0.86. Since the emotional loneliness subscale consists of six items and the social loneliness subscale consists of five items, the mean score per item has been used to measure emotional and social loneliness in the present study, in which we obtained Cronbach's alpha of 0.78 and 0.84 for emotional and social loneliness, respectively (refer to Table 4.2).

Cognitive Emotion Regulation Scale-Short (Garnefski et al., 2006). This short 18-item version of the Cognitive Emotion Regulation Questionnaire was developed by Garnefski and Kraaij (2006) from the 36-item version of the same questionnaire by Garnefski et al. (2001). The questionnaire has nine different conceptual subscales – self-blame, other-blame, rumination, catastrophizing, positive refocusing, planning, positive reappraisal, putting into perspective, and acceptance, with two items in each subscale. The scoring of this questionnaire is also based on a Likert scale, from 1 to 5, where 1 stands for "(almost) never," 2 signifies "sometimes," 3 stands for "regularly," and 4 and 5 signify "often" and "(almost) always," respectively. The scores of all nine different conceptual subscales were calculated separately and used to analyse the findings. According to Garnefski and Kraaij (2006), the alpha reliability of CERQ-Short subscales mostly ranged from 0.73 to 0.81. The validity of the tool is acceptably high. In the current study, Cronbach's alpha values ranged between 0.56 and 0.87 (refer to Table 4.2).

Data Collection and Study Setting

All data were collected with the help of an *online survey form* (Google forms), circulated among the participants via email and messaging applications, between 1st November 2020 and 30th November 2020, which was towards the end of the first wave of the COVID-19 pandemic in India. It was expected to take *approximately 15–20 minutes* to complete the survey. The participants took the survey after agreeing to the statement of consent given in the *informed consent form* provided at the beginning of the survey.

Examination, Scoring, and Statistical Analyses

After completion of data collection, the responses were scrutinized and scored. Since responding to all the items in the survey was necessary for submission, no incomplete response was received. It has already been stated that out of 135 responses, 17 were rejected due to reasons mentioned earlier. Hence, finally, data from 118 respondents (80 females and 38 males) were analysed. Scoring for all the scales was done by hand according to the manuals. The information schedule was coded, and a profile of the sample was drawn from it.

Then the statistical treatments of the scores were done by using *SPSS version 22.0*. Probability values to be accepted for the tests of significance were equal to or beyond 0.05 level. The statistical tools – mean, standard deviation, correlation, and hierarchical regression analysis – were selected following the objectives of the study after checking for all necessary assumptions. Also, since the study is exploratory in nature, after running the initial series of HMRAs as stated earlier, we selected those variables which significantly predicted global psychological well-being along with its different facets and rerun the HMRAs with them, an approach proposed by Field (2009). To determine whether the predictors accounted for a small, medium, or large amount of variance in well-being, we used Cohen's (1977) convention for small ($f^2 = 0.02$), medium ($f^2 = 0.15$), and large effects ($f^2 = 0.35$) as a standard.

Results

For the quantitative analyses, the data obtained from the subjects were systematically arranged and tabulated adequately for each of the variables considered in the present study. The data expressed as a measure of the variables constitute statistical distribution, and suitable techniques were used to analyse the distribution according to the earlier objectives.

The mean and standard deviation of all variables, that is the different components of loneliness, cognitive emotion regulation, and psychological well-being are depicted in Table 4.2.

Table 4.3 describes the correlation coefficients of the components of loneliness and cognitive emotion regulation with those of psychological well-being. The obtained findings revealed that both emotional and social lonelinesses were significantly and negatively related to global psychological well-being. A componential analysis suggested negative relationships of both types of lonelinesses to autonomy, environmental mastery, personal growth, and self-acceptance. However, the positive relations component is associated with social loneliness only.

Our findings further demonstrated that the adaptive cognitive emotion regulation strategies like positive reappraisal, planning, and putting into perspective were more strongly associated with higher levels of psychological well-being. Maladaptive strategies like catastrophizing, rumination, and self-blame were linked to poorer well-being, while acceptance, positive refocusing, and blaming others showed no or weaker association with well-being. Analysing the components, we found that refocus on planning and positive reappraisal were related to higher levels in all aspects of

Table 4.3 Pearson (r) correlation coefficients between different components of psychological well-being and those of the predictor variables: loneliness, cognitive emotion regulation, mindful self-care, and meaning in life (N = 118)

	Autonomy	Environmental Mastery	Personal Growth	Positive Relations	Purpose in Life	Self-Acceptance	Total PWB
Emotional Loneliness	-.333**	-.344**	-.182*	-0.161	-0.112	-.308**	-.337**
Social Loneliness	-.206*	-.414**	-.232*	-.344**	-0.144	-.335**	-.378**
Self-Blame	-.396**	-.218*	-0.125	0.014	-0.115	-.351**	-.297**
Acceptance	-0.012	-0.032	0.062	0.047	-0.043	-.204*	-0.054
Rumination	-.309**	-.208*	-.225*	-0.091	-0.092	-.374**	-.320**
Positive Refocusing	0.107	0.122	0.084	0.047	0.041	0.097	0.116
Planning	.210*	.252**	.364**	.185*	.345**	.245**	.367**
Positive Reappraisal	.326**	.418**	.511**	.206*	.217*	.489**	.516**
Putting into Perspective	0.057	.193*	.287**	.182*	0.098	.293**	.263**
Catastrophizing	-.425**	-.321**	-.402**	-.316**	-0.059	-.492**	-.485**
Other Blame	-0.016	-0.121	-0.025	-0.126	-0.051	-0.037	-0.077

PWB = Psychological Well-being
* $p < 0.05$; ** $p < 0.01$

Source: Author/s

psychological well-being. Putting into perspective showed positive relation-ships with four of the well-being components: environmental mastery, per-sonal growth, positive relations, and self-acceptance. Acceptance was found to be negatively correlated with the self-acceptance dimension. Autonomy, environmental mastery, and self-acceptance were negatively associated with self-blame. A relatively strong relationship was observed between cat-astrophizing and most psychological well-being dimensions except purpose in life. Rumination showed negative correlations with autonomy, environ-mental mastery, and self-acceptance. However, it is interesting to note here that positive refocusing and blaming others did not significantly correlate with any of the components of psychological well-being.

Hierarchical multiple regression analysis, as shown in Table 4.4, revealed that one or both components of loneliness were found to account for a significant amount of variance in global psychological well-being, along with most of its components except purpose in life. Including the relevant cognitive emotion regulation strategies in the subsequent models signifi-cantly explained additional variance beyond loneliness. While emotional and social loneliness explained 19.6% of the variance in total psychological well-being, inclusion of the components of cognitive emotion regulation in the model explained an additional 34.2% of the variance, emotional loneli-ness ($\beta = -0.142$), positive reappraisal ($\beta = 0.268$), planning ($\beta = 0.238$), self-blame ($\beta = -0.160$), and catastrophizing ($\beta = -0.245$) being the signifi-cant predictors. However, the models and relative contributions of the pre-dictors differed for the different components of psychological well-being.

For the individual facets, the significant predictors were: emotional lone-liness, self-blame, and catastrophizing for autonomy; emotional loneliness, social loneliness, positive reappraisal, and self-blame for environmental mastery; planning, positive reappraisal, and catastrophizing for personal growth; social loneliness and catastrophizing for positive relations; planning for purpose in life; positive reappraisal, putting into perspective, accept-ance, self-blame, rumination, and catastrophizing for self-acceptance.

Discussion

Predictive Role of Loneliness in Psychological Well-being

Our findings reveal that loneliness contributes to most of the dimen-sions of psychological well-being, except purpose in life. While the pre-vious literature shows loneliness as a negative predictor of well-being, the current study uniquely investigated the role of two types of loneli-nesses, as conceptualized by Weiss (1973), in predicting the different dimensions of psychological well-being (Ryff, 1989). Both emotional

Table 4.4 Hierarchical multiple regression analyses predicting global psychological well-being and its six components of loneliness and cognitive emotion regulation (N = 118)

Model	Criterion Variables	Predictor Variables	R^2	Adj. R^2	ΔR^2	$F\,(df_1,\,df_2)$	$\Delta F\,(df_1,\,df_2)$	Cohen's f^2 (R^2, ΔR^2)	β
1	Autonomy	Emotional loneliness	0.111	0.103	0.111	14.450*** (1, 116)	14.450*** (1, 116)	0.12, 0.12	-0.333***
2		Emotional loneliness	0.299	0.274	0.188	12.021*** (4, 113)	10.080*** (3, 113)	0.43, 0.23	-0.198*
		Self-blame							-0.230*
		Rumination							-0.080
		Catastrophizing							-0.276**
1	Environmental mastery	Emotional loneliness	0.222	0.208	0.222	16.369*** (2, 115)	16.369*** (2, 115)	0.29, 0.29	-0.237*
		Social loneliness							-0.339***
2		Emotional loneliness	0.327	0.303	0.106	13.744*** (4, 113)	8.877*** (2, 113)	0.49, 0.12	-0.178*
		Social loneliness							-0.251**
		Positive reappraisal							0.308***
		Self-blame							-0.155*
1	Personal growth	Social loneliness	0.054	0.046	0.054	6.594* (1, 116)	6.594* (1, 116)	0.05, 0.05	-0.232*
2		Social loneliness	0.368	0.345	0.314	18.694*** (3, 113)	16.423*** (4, 113)	0.58, 0.46	-0.036

Step	Predictor	Variable							β
		Planning							0.191*
		Positive reappraisal							0.323**
		Catastrophizing							-0.310***
1	Positive relations	Social loneliness	0.118	0.111	0.118	15.544*** (1, 116)	15.544*** (1, 116)	0.13, 0.13	-0.344***
2		Social loneliness	0.186	0.172	0.068	13.162*** (2, 115)	9.625** (1, 115)	0.23, 0.07	-0.299**
		Catastrophizing							-0.265**
1	Purpose in life	Planning	0.119	0.111	0.119	115.667*** (1, 116)	15.667*** (1, 116)	0.14, 0.14	0.345***
1	Self-acceptance	Emotional loneliness	0.158	0.143	0.158	10.764*** (2, 115)	10.764*** (2, 115)	0.19	-0.224*
		Social loneliness							-0.265**
2		Emotional loneliness	0.545	0.512	0.387	16.322*** (8, 109)	15.466*** (6, 109)	1.20, 0.63	-0.074
		Social loneliness							-0.122
		Positive reappraisal							0.306***
		Putting into perspective							0.207**
		Acceptance							-0.143*
		Self-blame							-0.210*
		Rumination							-0.196*
		Catastrophizing							-0.192*

(Continued)

Table 4.4 (Continued)

Model	Criterion Variables	Predictor Variables	R^2	Adj. R^2	ΔR^2	$F (df_1, df_2)$	$\Delta F (df_1, df_2)$	Cohen's f^2 (R^2, ΔR^2)	β
1	Global psychological well-being	Emotional loneliness	0.196	0.182	0.196	14.004*** (2, 115)	14.004*** (2, 115)	0.24	−0.242**
		Social loneliness							−0.302**
2		Emotional loneliness	0.538	0.509	0.342	18.293*** (7, 110)	16.286*** (5, 110)	1.16, 0.52	−0.143*
		Social loneliness							0.137
		Planning							0.238**
		Positive reappraisal							0.268**
		Self-blame							−0.160**
		Rumination							−0.143
		Catastrophizing							−0.245**

* $p < 0.05$; ** $p < 0.01$; ***$p < 0.001$

Source: Author/s

and social lonelinesses were significant predictors of global psychological well-being, along with the dimensions of environmental mastery and self-acceptance. Our results were consistent with recent findings revealing that loneliness negatively impacts overall psychological well-being (Shaheen et al., 2014) and related constructs like subjective vitality and psychological adjustment (Arslan, 2021). Other studies also reported that higher feelings of loneliness were associated with more psychological distress (Valiente et al., 2021) and poor emotional well-being (Stieger et al., 2021) during pandemic. Experiences of perceived social isolation due to "stay at home" orders were also found to be related to lower life satisfaction in adults (Clair et al., 2021).

Bruno (2000) also attributed the lack of social support and relationships to that of environmental mastery. In previous research, Thomas and Azmitia (2019) showed that individuals who reported spending time alone frequently but who did so for self-determined reasons appeared to be intrinsically motivated to spend time alone, displaying greater self-acceptance, as compared to their not self-determined counterparts (Thomas & Azmitia, 2019), a finding of much relevance in the context of the restrictions in commutation and social interaction prevalent at the time of the current study in India due to the pandemic.

The finding revealing emotional loneliness to be the single significant predictor of autonomy reiterated the proposition by Hirschfeld et al. (1977) that assertion of autonomy is one of the three cardinal dimensions of interpersonal dependency, along with emotional reliance on others and lack of social self-confidence. Our findings further demonstrated social loneliness as the single significant predictor of personal growth and positive relations. Though Moustakas (1961) suggested that loneliness can lead to personal growth and creativity through a confrontation or encounter with oneself, Osin and Leontiev (2013) were of a different opinion as they proposed a theoretical model of personal attitudes towards loneliness: acceptance and non-acceptance of loneliness, the facilitating and hindering the process of personal growth, respectively. Young adulthood is characterized as an age of forming social networks, and a chronic feeling of not being a part of a desired social network leads to an avoidance of solitude and to a continuous search for social contacts, which results in avoidance of self-encounter and becomes an obstacle for personal growth (Osin & Leontiev, 2013).

Results from this study are also consistent with the previous findings provided from the context of the COVID-19 pandemic (Serafini et al., 2020; Achdut & Refaeli, 2020). Although the concurrence of perceived loneliness with lower levels of psychological well-being in students has been observed even before the pandemic, in the current context, it may be attributed to the diverse losses associated with the halting of physical classes in educational institutions, such as the loss of sense of belonging, academics-related social interactions with peers and faculties, as well as those associated with curtailment in social interactions in other spheres of life and the support these interactions provide (Refaeli & Achdut, 2020).

Do Cognitive Emotion Regulation Strategies Add to the Predictive Utility in Psychological Well-being?

Findings from the present study indicate that cognitive emotion regulation strategies are essential in accounting for additional variances in global psychological well-being, along with each of its dimensions, after controlling for the impact of loneliness (see figures 4.1 to 4.7). Positive reappraisal and planning were obtained as significant positive predictors for global psychological well-being while catastrophizing and self-blame were significant negative predictors.

Role of Adaptive Strategies. Legerstee et al. (2011) proposed that the more one can use adaptive cognitive emotion regulation strategies, the better functioning state one's psyche usually is in. The current study revealed differential contributions of positive reappraisal, planning, and putting into perspective to the different dimensions of well-being. Positive reappraisal

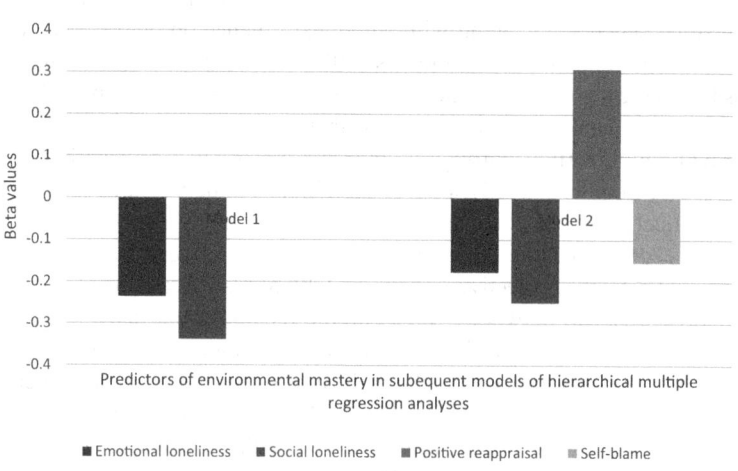

Figure 4.1 Graphical representation of beta values of the predictors of autonomy in the subsequent models of hierarchical multiple regression analyses

Source: Author/s

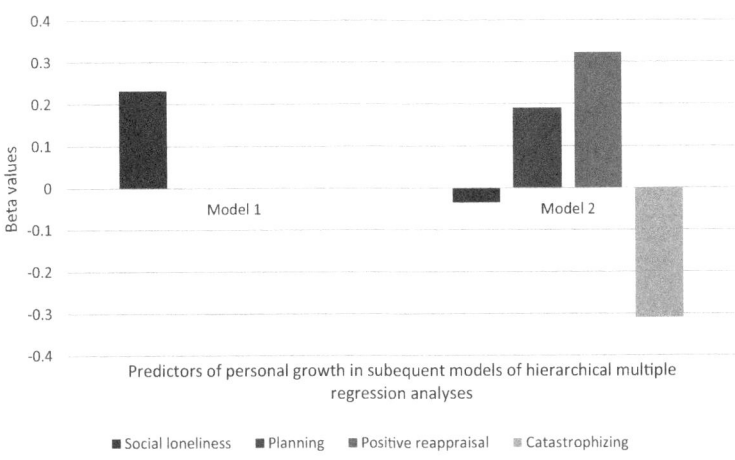

Figure 4.2 Graphical representation of beta values of the predictors of environmental mastery in the subsequent models of hierarchical multiple regression analyses

Source: Author/s

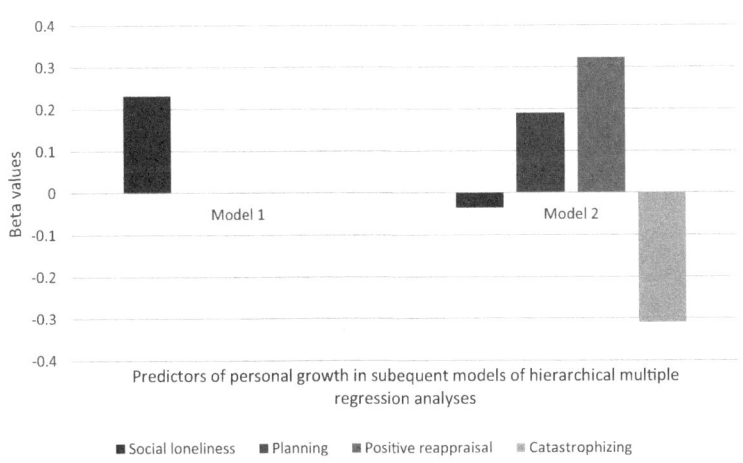

Figure 4.3 Graphical representation of beta values of the predictors of personal growth in the subsequent models of hierarchical multiple regression analyses

Source: Author/s

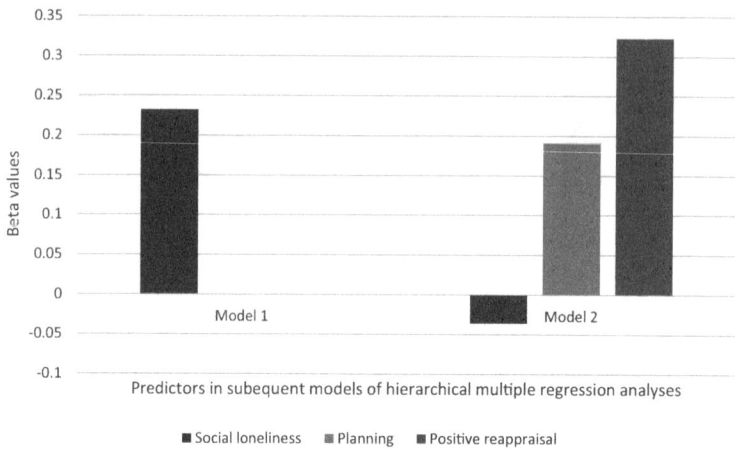

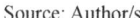

Figure 4.4 Graphical representation of beta values of the predictors of positive relations in the subsequent models of hierarchical multiple regression analyses

Source: Author/s

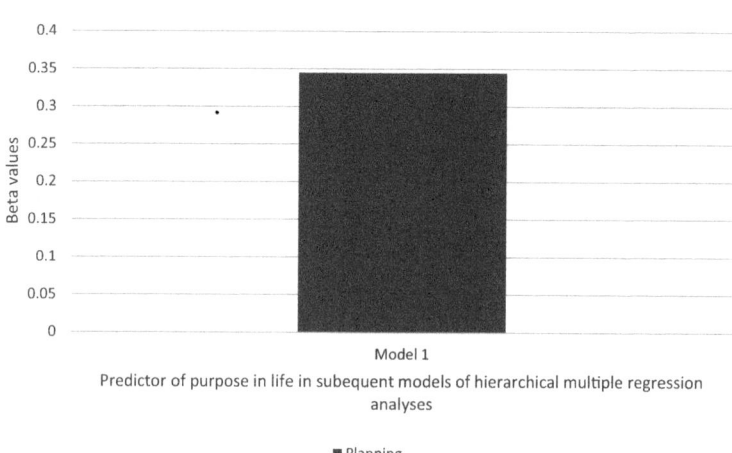

Figure 4.5 Graphical representation of beta values of the predictors of purpose in life in the subsequent models of hierarchical multiple regression analyses

Source: Author/s

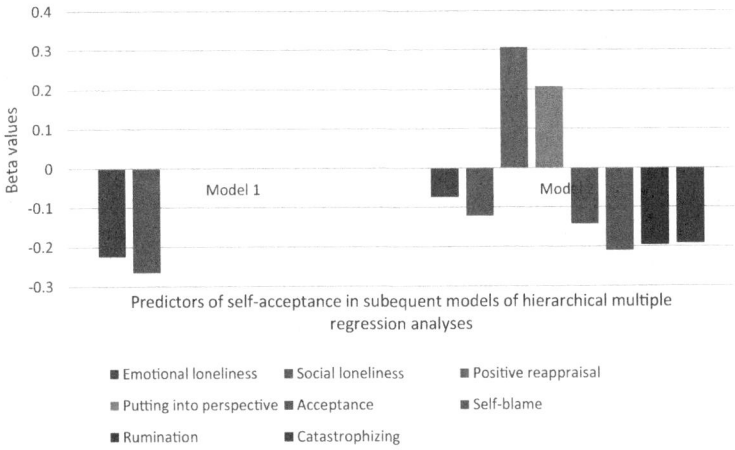

Figure 4.6 Graphical representation of beta values of the predictors of self-acceptance in the subsequent models of hierarchical multiple regression analyses

Source: Author/s

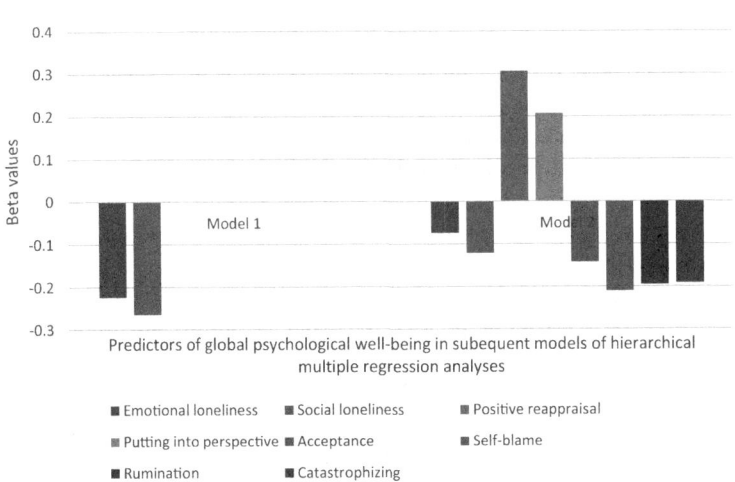

Figure 4.7 Graphical representation of beta values of the predictors of global psychological well-being in the subsequent models of hierarchical multiple regression analyses

Source: Author/s

is a cognitive process that involves focusing on the positive aspects of an adverse event, for instance, by reinterpreting the situation in terms of personal growth (Garnefski et al., 2001) leading to reduced distress (Garnefski & Kraaij, 2007), as well as to enhanced well-being (Karademas, 2007; Shiota, 2006). Planning may contribute to psychological well-being by facilitating goal attainment through directedness and self-determination (MacLeod & Conway, 2005). Again, being closely related to the concept of social comparison, putting into perspective involves thoughts of playing down the seriousness of the event or emphasizing its relativity when compared to other events and is an important issue concerning well-being (Janoff-Bulman, 1989). A recent study by Ruggieri and colleagues (2021) revealed that during the relatively later stages of COVID-19-related quarantine, online social comparison orientation may have fostered lower distress as well as greater life satisfaction and social connectedness, given that people felt that they were sharing the same difficult time, thus lessening the otherwise negative impact of social comparisons.

Role of Maladaptive Strategies. Among the maladaptive strategies, catastrophizing, self-blame, and rumination were found to account differentially for the variances of different well-being dimensions. In general, a catastrophizing style of coping is related to maladaptation, emotional distress, and depression (Sullivan et al., 1995) as well as to higher levels of negative mood and reduced personal growth in chronic pain and illness (Sturgeon & Zautra, 2013). Self-blame has been shown to be related to higher levels of depression (Anderson et al., 1994). In this context, Tedeschi (1999) reflects that blaming oneself may form an obstacle to adapting to unfavourable life events or trauma. In line with these theoretical underpinnings, our study also showed comparable findings. Being involved in experiencing repetitive thoughts in the absence of immediate environmental cueing (see Koole et al., 1999), although certain forms of ruminative thinking may help cope with stressful life events (Janoff-Bulman, 1989; Tedeschi, 1999), this thinking style, in general, is found to be related to depression (Nolen-Hoeksema, 2000; Nolen-Hoeksema et al., 1994, 1997), which is characterized by poor self-acceptance ability, also supported by the current results.

In the context of the current COVID-19 pandemic also, various studies have suggested a strong association between maladaptive cognitive emotion regulation strategies and poor psychological well-being outcomes in different populations. As pointed out by Restubog et al. (2020), making use of such strategies in dealing with the adverse situations that arise out of the context of the pandemic is indeed stressful. Dubey et al. (2020) also reported similar results in the Indian population during the pandemic. Further, another study by Wang et al. (2021) on Chinese nurses during the pandemic demonstrated significantly higher scores on the dimensions of rumination, self-blame, catastrophising, and other-blame, significantly lower scores on those of planning, positive refocus, and acceptance, in individuals with symptoms of depression or anxiety, in comparison to those without.

Integrating the Findings

The inclusion of cognitive emotion regulation strategies attenuated the impact of loneliness on global psychological well-being as well as its different dimensions. Unique sets of predictors were identified for global psychological well-being, and each of its individual facets, suggesting that differential combinations of psychological processes play pivotal roles in influencing the different components of psychological well-being. It seems clear from these results that although the components of loneliness and cognitive emotion regulation, in some way or another, show relationships with the facets of psychological well-being, the separate components refer to contributory or overlapping processes than to independent, disconnected components processes.

Limitations

However, the results of the present study need much caution in their interpretation and generalizability due to certain limiting factors such as the correlational, cross-sectional design and sample comprising a single age group from a single SES, counting only on self-report without including actual behavioural measures. Individuals suffering from clinical conditions were also not included in the study sample. Despite these limitations, the results have implications at different levels.

Implications

On a theoretical level, the present study contributes to the current body of literature about the determinants of the psychological well-being of students in their young adulthood. On the policy level, it underscores the importance of ensuring safe social interactions among students and instructors and fostering their ability to regulate emotions to promote their well-being. It also provides valuable insight into clinical interventions for individuals suffering from various chronic and acute psychological conditions in order not only to alleviate their psychological distress but to promote their psychological well-being as well, by aiding them to enhance their social connections and by incorporating various intentional emotion regulation strategies at the cognitive level of functioning to improve their overall lifestyle.

Conclusion

To conclude, both loneliness and cognitive emotion regulation play a cardinal role in contributing to the psychological well-being of Indian students. The present study further confirmed the multidimensionality and multi causality of psychological well-being by identifying unique sets of predictors for each facet. Most importantly, the current study indicates that intentionally engaging in cognitive processes of emotion regulation may function as potential strategies available to students for coping with the experience of chronic loneliness prevalent in the current times of restricted social interactions. This, in turn, would be instrumental in promoting their psychological well-being during and beyond the COVID-19 pandemic.

References

Anderson, C. A., Miller, R. S., Riger, A. L., Dill, J. C., & Sedikides, C. (1994). Behavioral and characterological attributional styles as predictors of depression and loneliness: Review, refinement, and test. *Journal of Personality and Social Psychology, 66*(3), 549.

Achdut, N., & Refaeli, T. (2020). Unemployment and psychological distress among young people during the COVID-19 pandemic: Psychological resources and risk factors. *International journal of environmental research and public health, 17*(19), 7163.

Arslan, G. (2021). Loneliness, college belongingness, subjective vitality, and psychological adjustment during coronavirus pandemic: Development of the College Belongingness Questionnaire. *Journal of Positive School Psychology, 5*(1), 17–31.

Ben-Zur, H. (2009). Coping styles and affect. *International Journal of Stress Management, 16*(2), 87.

Bruno, F. J. (2000). *Conquer Loneliness: menaklukkan kesepian.* Jakarta: PT Gramedia Pustaka Utama.

Clair, R., Gordon, M., Kroon, M., & Reilly, C. (2021). The effects of social isolation on well-being and life satisfaction during pandemic. *Humanities and Social Sciences Communications, 8*(1), 1–6.

Cohen, J. (1977). *Statistical power analysis for the behavioral sciences* (Rev. ed.). Academic Press.

Constantine, M. G., Okazaki, S., & Utsey, S. O. (2004). Self-concealment, social self-efficacy, acculturative stress, and depression in African, Asian, and Latin American international college students. *American Journal of Orthopsychiatry, 74*(3), 230–241.

De Jong-Gierveld, J., & Kamphuls, F. (1985). The development of a Rasch-type loneliness scale. *Applied Psychological Measurement, 9*(3), 289–299.

Dubey, N., Podder, P., & Pandey, D. (2020). Knowledge of COVID-19 and its influence on mindfulness, cognitive emotion regulation and psychological flexibility in the Indian community. *Frontiers in Psychology, 11*, 3031.

Ferguson, N., Laydon, D., Nedjati Gilani, G., Imai, N., Ainslie, K., Beguelin, M., Bhatia, S., Boonyasiri, A., Cucunubá, Z., Cuomo-Dannenburg, G., Dighe, A., Dorigatti, I., Fu, H., Gaythorpe, K., Green, W., Hamlet, A., Hinsley, W., Okell, L. C., van Elsland, S., . . . Ghani, A. (2020). *Report 9: Impact of non-pharmaceutical interventions (NPIs) to reduce COVID-19 mortality and healthcare demand.* https://spiral.imperial.ac.uk/handle/10044/1/77482

Field, A. (2009). *Discovering statistics using SPSS* (3rd ed.). Sage Publications.

Garnefski, N., Kraaij, V., & Spinhoven, P. (2001). Negative life events, cognitive emotion regulation and emotional problems. *Personality and Individual differences, 30*(8), 1311–1327.

Garnefski, N., & Kraaij, V. (2006). Cognitive emotion regulation questionnaire–development of a short 18-item version (CERQ-short). *Personality and Individual Differences, 41*(6), 1045–1053.

Garnefski, N., & Kraaij, V. (2007). The cognitive emotion regulation questionnaire. *European Journal of Psychological Assessment, 23*(3), 141–149.

Gross, J. J. (2001). Emotion regulation in adulthood: Timing is everything. *Current Directions in Psychological Science, 10*(6), 214–219.

Gross, J. J., & John, O. P. (2003). Individual differences in two emotion regulation processes: Implications for affect, relationships, and wellbeing. *Journal of Personality and Social Psychology, 85*(2), 348.

Gupta, K., & Parimal, B. S. (2020). Relationship between personality dimensions and psychological wellbeing among university students during pandemic lockdown. *Journal of Global Resources, 6*(01a). https://doi.org/10.46587/JGR.2020.v06si01.002

Holmes, E. A., O'Connor, R. C., Perry, V. H., Tracey, I., Wessely, S., Arseneault, L., Ballard, C. G., Christensen, H., Cohen Silver, R., Everall, I., Ford, T., John, A., Kabir, T., King, K., Madan, I., Michie, S., Przybylski, A. K., Shafran, R., Sweeney, A., . . . Bullmore, E. (2020). Multidisciplinary research priorities for the COVID-19 pandemic: A call for action for mental health science. *The Lancet Psychiatry, 7*(6), 547–560. https://doi.org/10.1016/S2215-0366(20)30168-1

Hirschfeld, R. M., Klerman, G. L., Gouch, H. G., Barrett, J., Korchin, S. J., & Chodoff, P. (1977). A measure of interpersonal dependency. *Journal of personality assessment, 41*(6), 610-618.

Janoff-Bulman, R. (1989). Assumptive worlds and the stress of traumatic events: Applications of the schema construct. *Social cognition, 7*(2), 113.

Karademas, E. C. (2007). Positive and negative aspects of wellbeing: Common and specific predictors. *Personality and Individual Differences, 43*, 277–287.

Keyes, C. L. (2002). The mental health continuum: From languishing to flourishing in life. *Journal of Health and Social Behavior*, 207–222. https://doi.org/10.2307/3090197

Koole, S. L., Smeets, K., Van Knippenberg, A., & Dijksterhuis, A. (1999). The cessation of rumination through self-affirmation. *Journal of Personality and Social Psychology, 77*(1), 111.

Luhman, M., & Hawkley, L. C. (2016). Age differences in loneliness from late adolescence to oldest-old age. *Developmental Psychology, 52*, 943–959.

Legerstee, J. S., Garnefski, N., Verhulst, F. C., & Utens, E. M. (2011). Cognitive coping in anxiety-disordered adolescents. *Journal of adolescence, 34*(2), 319–326.

MacLeod, A. K., & Conway, C. (2005). Well-being and the anticipation of future positive experiences: The role of income, social networks, and planning ability. *Cognition & emotion, 19*(3), 357–374.

Moustakas, C. (1961). The sense of self. *Journal of Humanistic Psychology, 1*(1), 20–34.

Nolen-Hoeksema, S. (2000). The role of rumination in depressive disorders and mixed anxiety/depressive symptoms. *Journal of Abnormal Psychology, 109*(3), 504.

Nolen-Hoeksema, S., McBride, A., & Larson, J. (1997). Rumination and psychological distress among bereaved partners. *Journal of Personality and Social Psychology, 72*(4), 855.

Nolen-Hoeksema, S., Parker, L. E., & Larson, J. (1994). Ruminative coping with depressed mood following loss. *Journal of Personality and Social Psychology, 67*(1), 92.

Osin, E., & Leontiev, D. (2013). Multidimensional inventory of loneliness experience: Structure and properties. *Psychology. Journal of Higher School of Economics, 10*(1), 55–81.

Refaeli, T., & Achdut, N. (2020). Perceived poverty, perceived income adequacy and loneliness in Israeli young adults: Are social capital and neighbourhood capital resilience factors? *Health & Social Care in the Community, 30*(2).

Restubog, S. L. D., Ocampo, A. C. G., & Wang, L. (2020). Taking control amidst the chaos: Emotion regulation during the COVID-19 pandemic. *Journal of Vocational Behavior, 119.*

Ruggieri, S., Ingoglia, S., Bonfanti, R. C., & Coco, G. L. (2021). The role of online social comparison as a protective factor for psychological wellbeing: A longitudinal study during the COVID-19 quarantine. *Personality and Individual Differences, 171,* 110486.

Ryan, R. M., & Deci, E. L. (2001). On happiness and human potentials: A review of research on hedonic and eudaimonic wellbeing. *Annual Review of Psychology, 52*(1), 141–166.

Ryff, C. D. (1989). Happiness is everything, or is it? Explorations on the meaning of psychological wellbeing. *Journal of Personality and Social Psychology, 57*(6), 1069.

Seligman, M. E., & Csikszentmihalyi, M. (2014). Positive psychology: An introduction. In *Flow and the foundations of positive psychology* (pp. 279–298). Springer.

Serafini, G., Parmigiani, B., Amerio, A., Aguglia, A., Sher, L., & Amore, M. (2020). The psychological impact of COVID-19 on the mental health in the general population. *QJM: An International Journal of Medicine, 113*(8), 531–537.

Shaheen, F., & Jahan, M. (2014). Role of social support in combating psychological distress among senior secondary school students. *Indian Journal of Positive Psychology, 5*(2), 163.

Shiota, M. (2006). Silver linings and candles in the dark: Differences among positive coping strategies in predicting subjective wellbeing. *Emotion, 6,* 335–339.

Stieger, S., Lewetz, D., & Swami, V. (2021). Emotional well-being under conditions of lockdown: An experience sampling study in Austria during the COVID-19 pandemic. *Journal of Happiness Studies*, 1–18.

Sturgeon, J. A., & Zautra, A. J. (2013). Psychological resilience, pain catastrophizing, and positive emotions: Perspectives on comprehensive modeling of individual pain adaptation. *Current Pain and Headache Reports, 17*(3), 317.

Sullivan, M. J., Bishop, S. R., & Pivik, J. (1995). The pain catastrophizing scale: Development and validation. *Psychological Assessment, 7*(4), 524.

Tedeschi, R. G. (1999). Violence transformed: Posttraumatic growth in survivors and their societies. *Aggression and Violent Behavior, 4*(3), 319–341.

Thomas, V., & Azmitia, M. (2019). Motivation matters: Development and validation of the motivation for solitude scale–short form (MSS-SF). *Journal of Adolescence, 70*, 33–42.

Valiente, C., Contreras, A., Peinado, V., Trucharte, A., Martínez, A. P., & Vázquez, C. (2021). Psychological adjustment in Spain during the COVID-19 pandemic: Positive and negative mental health outcomes in the general population. *The Spanish Journal of Psychology, 24*.

Van Bavel, J. J., Baicker, K., Boggio, P. S., Capraro, V., Cichocka, A., Cikara, M., Crockett, M. J., Crum, A. J., Douglas, K. M., Druckman, J. N., Drury, J., Dube, O., Ellemers, N., Finkel, E. J., Fowler, J. H., Gelfand, M., Han, S.,Haslam, S. A., Jetten, J., . . . Willer, R. (2020). Using social and behavioural science to support COVID-19 pandemic response. *Nature Human Behaviour, 4*(5), 460–471. https://doi.org/10.1038/s41562-020-0884-z

Wang, Q. Q., Fang, Y. Y., Huang, H. L., Lv, W. J., Wang, X. X., Yang, T. T., Yuan, J. M., Gao, Y., Qian, R. L., & Zhang, Y. H. (2021). Anxiety, depression and cognitive emotion regulation strategies in Chinese nurses during the COVID-19 outbreak. *Journal of Nursing Management, 29*(5).

Weiss, R. S. (1973). *Loneliness: The experience of emotional and social isolation.* MIT Press.

5 Nobody's Child

Managing Mental Trauma of Children With Mental Health Issues

Aniruddha Deb

Introduction

The unprecedented crises created by the COVID-19 in the global Mental Health sphere are yet ill understood, and it has been speculated that it will take decades for us to appropriately evaluate the devastation that has been wreaked upon the population all over the world. Information gleaned from surveys that have been undertaken by various agencies at a preliminary level indicates that for around half the population of the world, the pandemic and resultant lockdown procedures have resulted in a negative effect on our Mental Health. The director-general of International Committee of the Red Cross (ICRC) Robert Mardini said: "The COVID-19 health crisis has exacerbated the psychological distress of millions of people. Lockdown restrictions, a loss of social interaction, and economic pressures are all impacting people's Mental Health and access to care." (WHO, 2021)

When we assess the impact of COVID-19 on the Mental Health of people, we can subdivide the issues into three categories: 1) People who had no Mental Health issues at all, yet the pandemic has made them mentally ill or at least has had deleterious effects on their mental status; 2) those who had potential or underlying Mental Health issues that were exposed or exacerbated into a diagnosable Mental Health condition; and 3) those with existing Mental Health issues and/or diagnosis, who were affected negatively in more than one way. Reduced access to Mental Health care has been a bane for many— if not all, access to psychiatrists, psychologists, and other Mental Health care workers has been remarkably limited to say the least. Procuring medication had become difficult for a large number of patients—especially in the remote areas, and social restrictions took a toll on many more (WHO, 2021).

Compounded with this were the factors of fear and anxiety, loneliness due to social isolation, living in a bubble, redundancy, and other financial pressures that caused a lot of difficulties for families around the world (WHO, 2021).

Common difficulties faced by every child with a Mental Health issue have included both the direct and the indirect effects. The fact that children are not

DOI: 10.4324/9781003348429-5

allowed to go to school is having effects on their academics, their social inter-actions, and play – which in turn are affecting their cognitive development, neuromuscular coordination, and sports abilities. Similarly, lack of commu-nication, interactive play and games, team sports, and so on is going to have long-lasting effects on their interactive abilities – their performance in group situations, team-activities, and bonding together at work and play. The par-ents and other caregivers of these children are going through the same Men-tal Health issues as stated before. The adult interactions in the house and the lack or over-zealous caregiving with the children at home round the clock for months on end can have untold effects on their growing psyche and Mental Health which our science and literature have had no scope to study in the past.

Children with Mental Health issues – what is happening in lockdown?

In spite of the high levels of co-variations between the categories, chil-dren with Mental Health issues are commonly pigeonholed as having either "externalizing" or "internalizing" disorders. Externalizing disorders are understood to be characterized by problematic behaviour related to poor impulse control, including rule breaking, aggression, impulsivity, and inattention. Specific child and adolescent externalizing disorders include conduct disorder (Sameck & Hicks, 2014). Internalizing disorders, on the other hand, are most often characterized by quiet, internal distress some-times referred to as "intropunitive," rather than overtly, socially negative, or disruptive behaviour. Such features may also make these disorders more difficult to detect in the very young who have less well-developed verbal skills in general and specifically an even more limited capacity to describe internal feeling states (Tandon et al., 2009).

It is evident that children with either kind of disorder will react differently to any difficulty that they might face. Children with externalizing disorders are likely to react behaviourally, while children with internalizing disorders will react with quiet distress, the extent of which is often not very evident to the non-perspicacious observer.

Not all effects have been empirically studied – indeed, the situation has not remained the same, and parameters have shifted. Not everyone has been impacted equally. Some families have faced bereavement – a few have lost many close relatives and friends, some have faced loss of job —some are in dire financial distress, some have had to leave their places of residence and travel to their sites of origin, yet others have had no such calamity visiting them, their families have not faced any major crisis – only the inconven-ience of not being able to go out as they please and being cooped up in the same household which may or may not be adequately spacious for the number of dwellers remain the common element.

Children with externalizing disorders

Parents of children with attention deficit disorder (ADD) have sought professional help from nearly the initiation of the lockdown. Recognizing that children with ADD are particularly vulnerable to the distress caused by the pandemic and physical distancing measures, and they might display increased behavioural problems, associated with the additional difficulty on the part of the clinician to deliver care within the new restrictions, the European ADHD Guidelines Group (EAGG) has developed guidance on the assessment and management of ADHD during the COVID-19 virus pandemic. Given the requirement for physical distancing, it has been recommended that all relevant service provision should continue via telephone or some other appropriate online video technology, in line with current recommendations for the use of telepsychiatry within the framework of the law of the land and/or recommendations from highly regarded agencies such as the UK Royal College of Psychiatrists or the American Psychiatric Association. It was recommended that schools and teachers should try to monitor all their students but should include those with ADHD, especially adolescents, as a priority group, because of their disorganisation and increased level of risk. For example are they participating in online classes, and are they submitting their tasks? Are there concerns about their social and emotional well-being?

For families with ADD children, the EAGG recommends the use of behavioural parenting strategies because they improve parenting and have beneficial effects in reducing oppositional defiant and disruptive behaviour, which is common in ADHD. Parents were encouraged to seek self-help versions of evidence-based systems, who were wary of trying out untested methods easily available in today's information-overload methods such as the questionable websites on the Internet. The Lancet's recommendations are easily and freely available on the Internet—especially the supplementary appendix to the June, 2020 issue for further study and application (Cortese et al., 2020). They will be discussed in some greater detail in the management section, vide infra.

The EAGC has further recommended that children with ADHD should either continue or can be started on medication for management of the condition—that medication should not be held back in consideration of the fact that we are in a lockdown situation due to the pandemic and that schools and other teaching institutions are not open yet. Behaviour related to ADHD can become more disorganised and disruptive in these unsupervised and poorly controlled times. Also, this in turn is likely to compromise the maintenance of COVID-19 protocol – such as maintaining physical distancing and avoiding going out unless essential. On the other hand, parents and caregivers have been requested not to increase or add doses to the prescribed medication, however much it might be tempting to curb excesses with medication. As it is, the state of lockdown was not conducive to procuring medication – though it has been seen that restricted chemicals have been made available more easily by both government regulation and other means (Cortese et al., 2020).

Finally, the EAGC has also recommended that while on the one hand children should neither be controlled with antipsychotics, on the other, nor should drug holidays be planned—since situations like lockdown, where parents are perforce having to spend large number of hours indoors with ADHD children, are more likely to exacerbate symptoms than not.

A recent study published from Bangladesh (Mallick and Radwan, 2021) has looked into various Mental Health issues across mentally ill children of various diagnoses. The authors found that when compared with the period prior to lockdown, the prevalence of emotional disorder, conduct disorder, and hyperactivity had increased significantly during the lockdown period. Conduct disorder and hyperactivity were more prevalent among boys both before and within lockdown. In contrast, prevalence of emotional disorder was higher among girls before lockdown, but within the lockdown period, the boy-girl prevalence was almost the same. In fact, in both boys and girls, conduct disorder had approximately doubled during lockdown as compared with the period prior to lockdown.

This same study has commented that ADHD has been found to be increased to almost three-fold during lockdown. A lot of symptoms of ADHD can be explained by the boredom of daily life during lockdown and the inability of virtual classrooms to provide adequate academic milieu to millions of youngsters.

Children with internalizing disorders

With anxiety and depression having become the neo-"normal," it is not surprising that the same picture has been seen in the youngsters too. The Weil Institute for Neurosciences, University of California, San Francisco, in a document published in early 2021 (Emotional Well-Being and Coping During COVID-19) has welcomed the anxiety because it has helped us cope, bond together from a distance due to the pandemic norms, and thus slow the spread of the virus. The anxiety, even if it is uncomfortable, has thus been termed "a good thing" now.

The pandemic has put children across the world in an unenviable position of not being able to attend school any more. By April 2020, schools in 188 countries have been suspended, putting 90% of the enrolled learners (1.5 billion people) out of education (UNESCO). In the case of children with special needs and mentally ill children, this has put extra burden. A lot of facilities are extended to children through schools. In a survey by the Mental Health charity YoungMinds, which included 2111 participants up to age 25 years with a mental illness history in the UK, 83% said the pandemic had made their conditions worse. Twenty-six per cent said they were unable to access Mental Health support; peer support groups and face-to-face services have been cancelled, and support by phone or online can be challenging for some young people. As it is, parents are finding it difficult to manage to get children to concentrate on their work for long enough— compounded with anxiety or depression, the problem becomes manifold, since both depression and anxiety erode focusing and concentration abilities.

Routines are important for children with depression to cope with the stress of day-to-day life. Inability to go to school has caused severe worsening of depression in many children. There have been anecdotal records of children locking themselves up in their rooms for days on end, not coming out – often not bathing, eating, or even leaving their beds (Lancet, 2020). Just as it has been difficult for them during the pandemic, it will be similarly difficult for children with depression to restart regular schooling after the restrictions are reduced and schooling restarts.

One category of children with internalizing Mental Health issues are children with obsessive compulsive disorder (OCD). OCD is strongly associated with anxiety, and because COVID-19 protocol insists on ritualized hand washing, too, such children will get a double dose of increase in anxiety features and obsessions.

In a study by Nissen et al. (2020), authors have described worsening of their OCD, anxiety, and depressive symptoms in two groups of children (children/adolescents newly diagnosed at a specialized OCD clinic and a survey group identified through the Danish OCD Association). The worsening was more pronounced in the survey group. Aggravation of OCD correlated with the worsening of anxiety, depressive symptoms, and the extent of avoidance behaviour. For both groups, OCD aggressive symptoms predicted a significant worsening. Poor baseline insight showed a trend to predict a symptom worsening. The worsening was most pronounced in children with an early age of onset and a family history of attention deficit hyperactivity disorder.

In a narrative review by Vittoria Zaccari et al. (2021), two out of three studies on children and adolescents showed an exacerbation of OCD and a worsening even in the presence of an ongoing treatment.

Children with developmental disorders

Developmental disorders primarily include autism spectrum disorders and mental retardation. This category includes children with learning issues who need structure and rigorous methods of learning and constant inputs from special educators, psychologists, occupation therapists, etc., for adequate and appropriate achievement of developmental levels. The prolonged effects of lockdown and staying away from school are already having their deleterious effects on this population. Children are being brought to clinics with regressing milestones, increased activity levels, difficulty in management, sleep and eating patterns—indeed, the whole plethora of behavioural issues are skyrocketing due to the restrictions imposed upon the child–adolescent with special needs—parents are at their wits' end to understand how to best handle the needs of special children when there is no school, special education system, and, indeed, individual special educators available for day-to-day guidance and management.

Children with autism have had a difficult time in the last nearly 2 years. Difficulty in processing new information, changes in daily routine, new routine, or activities – all tend to distress them. It has all happened in the period of lockdown during the pandemic. Consequently, social communication has reduced, unsupervised time has increased, and stereotyped behaviour patterns have increased as a consequence. New rules of COVID-19-protocol had to be taught and learnt – repetitive questions have had to be faced. As the lockdown rules were relaxed, even newer rules had to be followed – as a consequence new behavioral problems and repetitive behaviour had to be fended off again.

Management of Children with Mental Health diagnoses during COVID-19 pandemic and Lockdown

In children with externalizing disorders: Management of boredom, excessive energy within the confines of home environment, and engagement in academics with relatively less supervision will have to be the focus. The EAGG recommends the use of behavioural parenting strategies because they improve parenting and have beneficial effects in reducing oppositional defiant and disruptive behaviour, which is common in ADHD (Cortese et al., 2020). The same can be extrapolated to children and adolescents with CD and other disruptive behavior disorders. Recommendations from the EAGC guiding parents in confinement during the COVID-19 crisis adapted from "How to . . . parent under pressure" include strategies such as

1. Staying positive and motivated, 2. Making sure all family members know what is expected of them, 3. Building your child's self-confidence and trust in you, 4. Helping your child to follow instructions, 5. Promoting better behaviour; and 6. Limiting conflicts (Cortese et al., 2020). These recommendations have helped countless parents and guardians across the world, but the actual application is not without its challenges.

In children with internalizing disorders: The primary issues that need management in the handling of children and adolescents during the

COVID-19 time are as follows: anxiety, depression, boredom, obsessions—depending upon the mental challenges the child is facing. Anxiety is an issue that has to be handled in every child (and indeed, adult) to manage the effects that COVID-19 is having on the minds of the entire population. Anxiety has its own way of playing out – in the beginning of the pandemic, there was widespread anxiety in a certain section of the population, worries about getting infected, and the consequences of the infection. People were afraid of people, took elaborate measures of disinfecting themselves, others, objects, and, in some cases, even the food that they were going to cook and eat. Gradually, as information came in regarding the nature of spread of the SARS-CoV-2 virus, people became more pragmatic, but by that time they had begun to feel the negative effects of lack of social interaction in the conventional manner, wanted to go out of their homes, and lead a "normal" life. Children have been no different from this.

One of the direct consequences of this kind of anxiety—at first of the illness and then the restrictions imposed by the illness—was a paranoia of others which was not truly psychotic in nature. However, a study involving more than 2,000 participants in five countries (Norway, Germany, Brazil, Columbia, and Israel) in the two waves in April and July 2020 indicated that paranoia did not increase as would have been expected – despite a significant increase in the level of distress among the respondents (Mækelæ et al., 2021).

Similar studies involving children are probably lacking, though organizations like the "Child Mind Institute" have warned about paranoia in children that might be "passed on by worried parents."

The first several months, however, have been increasingly difficult for children and adolescents who have suffered silently in the confines of their houses, very often in company of grown-ups in situations where they have not been part of most, if at all, of grown-up conversations. More than one child has felt that their months in lockdown was spent "in watching the same four walls of the house, the same two faces of the parents (who say the same things) and the same tree outside the window." This lack of variety – something we take so much for granted in our daily lives has had tremendous deleterious effects on the cognition and psyche of the growing minds – like after the Spanish flu epidemic, or the Holocaust, the aftermath of this pandemic and lockdown is likely to haunt the human civilization for at least decades after it is over.

Experts have repeatedly, in the lay press and on academic platforms, suggested ways to counter the anxiety and depression in these situations. Those who have followed these have invariably felt improvement in their mental status and been more relieved than they were beforehand. One of the first rules of stress management is to remove oneself from the source of the stress. In this case, a lot of the stress have generated from the news pertaining to the events surrounding the pandemic. I use the word "news" with reservation. While actual news services could not provide news that built confidence and gave relief, one accepts that it was difficult in the early parts of the pandemic, as the parallel source of information – the social media – did great harm in both highlighting the negatives and providing extra sources of anxiety and tension by highlighting the horrible, and also by flooding the platform with fake and untrue news. When it is not easy to differentiate between the "right" and the "wrong," it is better to avoid both rather than even spend several hours in trying to see what is true and correct. Other methods of keeping well are to take care of the physical health – deep breaths, stretching, or meditation; eating healthy, well-balanced meals exercising regularly, sleeping adequately and avoiding excessive alcohol, tobacco, and substance use; making time to unwind – try to do some other enjoyable activities; connecting with others – talking to trustworthy people about concerns and feelings; connecting with the community or faith-based organizations – even while maintaining social distancing measures. Involving the older child and adolescent in this kind of activity also gives them a sense of purpose, not feeling as if they are wasting their days doing nothing. Helping others cope is also a strong way of feeling empowered and validating one's purpose in life. For further reading, the US Centre for Disease Control (National Center for Chronic Disease Prevention and Health Promotion, Division of Population Health) has a wealth of information on their website.

Not all, but many children and adolescents with depression and anxiety will require regular psychotherapy due to the stress of life in the pandemic times. While it is not easy to travel to the therapist's clinic/office, it is now necessary to accept the online therapeutic modes –by virtual video calling. One appreciates that on the one hand every activity has become screen based and online, causing pedagogues to worry about the increased and near constant screen-time for children, it is also now a necessary evil which we have to accept to manage the pandemic situation.

Children with developmental disorders: Children with ASD will need time to process the information related to the pandemic. By the time this book sees the light of day, the world would have moved on from the complete lockdown and home-bound situation that we had found ourselves at the end of the first quarter of 2020. Yet, life will still be very different from the pre-COVID-19 era, and, undoubtedly, more and more changes – most of which will be in moving towards "normal" – will be in place, while a lot of "neo-normal" rules will be with us to stay. While the entire population will have to continuously adjust, children with ASD will find it difficult to go through this series of changes. Very often, social stories help children with autism to adjust to new situations and develop this knowledge. The UNICEF has developed such social stories which are available on their websites.

One of the problems that parents and guardians have faced with children with ASD is that they have obsessively asked questions repeatedly about the COVID-19 virus, COVID-19, the pandemic, and lockdown. Reacting with anger and frustration is easy, but it does not help the situation. Many pedagogues have recommended the use of "time windows" for this kind of activity. A certain time period – for example half an hour or so – is allotted to "question-hour" when all questions about the issue is addressed – but at other times, such questions are not allowed. Attempts to include the COVID-19 virus in the play routine of the child should be allowed – this helps in managing the stress due to the issue.

Home education of children with autism has been found to be helpful. In a Filipino study, (Cahapay, 2020) five themes have emerged in this experience that parents have had during the lockdown.

Theme 1: many are better than one in home education during isolation. While therapeutic services were nearly inaccessible, families pooled their own resources together and found that many hands make light work – while in actuality, some members may be better in handling certain issues (e.g. father may be better at teaching, elder brother in engaging in non-academic activities, and mother in managing temper tantrums).

Theme 2: from struggles with the transition to cultivation of new activities – parents struggled in the beginning to manage the children, but later realized that there can be activities without involving the computer where children can participate – and be happy.

Theme 3: new social reality in preparation for the post-pandemic period – most parents have spent this time in educating their children with special needs the meaning of a new, post-pandemic world – the deserted streets due to COVID-19 lockdown, the need for distancing, or masking and most importantly – the new rules of socialization in the post-pandemic period.

Theme 4: all forms of home education are essential – home education provides for optimal learning.

Theme 5: families encouraging families in these tough times. A family that has a child with autism is a part of a larger family of children with autism. Other parents offer tips on how to teach their children with autism adapt to the new situation. All types of encouragement from other families and the community are essential in the home education for children with autism. When there is a presence of encouragement among families, it is more likely to be from other families who have the same experiences. However, due to restrictions brought by the COVID-19 situation, families may be alone in managing their children with autism. Narzisi (2020), suggested maintaining online contact with the therapists, teachers, caregivers, and other parents to share and gain different types of support needed for the continued education of children with autism at home. The same author has also suggested a ten-step programme for helping caregivers cope with children of autism in this period of the pandemic.

They include 1. Explaining to your child what COVID-19 is, 2. Structuring daily life activities, 3. Handling semi-structured play activities, 4. Using serious games (to improve social cognition and to recognize facial emotions, emotional gestures, and emotional situations), 5. Sharing video game and/or Internet sessions with parents, 6. Implementing and sharing special interests with parents, 7. Online therapy for high-functioning children, 8. Online consultations for parents and caregivers, 9. Maintaining contact with the school, and 10. Leaving spare time for doing nothing (or maybe take a walk around the house).

We must win the war against the COVID-19 virus and emerge unscathed to continue as a civilized species on Earth. Every one of us is a part of this battle, and we must learn to educate ourselves, manage our emotions, and create scopes for others in society for handling this extraordinary and bizarre horror that is not restricted to the movie theatre or the screen of our living rooms. Small battles have been lost or won, a lot have been learnt – unfortunately through the loss of many lives – but we seem to be turning the tide, at least in some areas. We need to be pragmatic, and our efforts must not abate. Only then will we be able to completely turn the tide in this current global crisis.

Stress in children in a post-COVID-19 world

Although we have not emerged entirely from the pandemic and its effects, we are already experiencing the aftermath in all population segments of a post-COVID-19 world. Children who have been born in the beginning of the pandemic are around 2 years old now. Children who were going to school has had a 2-year layoff. Peer relations have not built up in children who should have started playing in playgrounds, interacted with others in Montessories and other schools. Teachers are reporting an inordinate increase in anxiety in children of all ages in our clinics, even grown up children are worried about going back to school, interacting with teachers, and other students. The effects of enforced loneliness on the growth and development of children, the resulting deleterious effects on children's cognitive functions due to reduced arborization owing to the enforced isolation for 2 years and more are yet to be studied, but there is no doubt that socialization has an important role to play in brain development and academics (Blakemore, 2010).

In a recent open-access article presented online by Braj Bhushan et al. (2022), studies have been quoted in China that have found more than 10% children and adolescents in a large (15,993) cohort aged 8 to 18 years, meeting the criteria of PTS. The same article quotes a larger (28.5%) prevalence in Turkey. Most of these studies found a higher prevalence in rural areas – the possible reason being that in rural areas, infrastructure to manage COVID-19 was lacking in most countries (Bhushan et al., 2022). Severe shortage of medication, hospital beds, and oxygen in India; the Mental Health toll due to the process of hospitalization itself; struggles to reach medical facilities, financial issues, coupled with the constant fear of losing a loved one, all have had severe effects on the population. The authors have noted that features of PTS were interestingly more prominent in individuals who did not lose a near relative in the pandemic than those who did. The reason offered is that the "slow deterioration of health", along with the "expectation of worst outcome" actually allowed participants to reach acceptance than those who did not.

One of the crucial aspects of this study (Bhushan et al., 2022) was the finding that those who were exposed to electronic media had greater PTS than those who did not. The same effect of the print media was not observed. The possible reasons were the over-exposure to videos of "people running to hospitals, mass burials, burning pyres, the crying faces, and other horrific scenes." Also, exposure to material available on the electronic media could be repetitive and for longer periods than with the print media.

Positive psychological changes (Post Traumatic Growth – PTG) have also been reported in this phase. In the future, more studies will show us how our children are faring as our world comes out further from this recent horror that humanity has gone through.

Conclusion

The world has not yet seen the end of COVID-19 or SARS-CoV-2. However, as the spate of infection, hospitalization, and death abates, we are limping back to what we used to know as being normal. A new world is emerging, and more of this newness is yet waiting to be discovered. Children are developing differently, parents are unable to provide the necessary psychological and social support, there is hardly any peer interaction yet, and adults in their lives are too preoccupied with their own distresses to give the kind of support a growing child needs. In many situations, children are being allowed to almost fend for themselves in social and familial areas and in the area of cognitive development and these will surely show their true colours in the years to come.

On a positive note, the nearly-post-COVID-19 world has witnessed children displaying an array of coping mechanisms leading to PTG. It is heartening to note that the human psyche has the ability to overcome distress and disaster and forge ahead in a positive manner.

References

5 ways the COVID-19 pandemic has impacted mental health. (2021, May 18). *Wellbeing.* https://www.who.int/europe/emergencies/situations/covid-19/mental-health-and-covid-19

Bhushan, B., Basu, S., & Ganai, U. J. (2022). Post-traumatic stress and growth among the children and adolescents in the aftermath of COVID-19. *Frontiers in Psychology, 12.* https://doi.org/10.3389/fpsyg.2021.791263

Blakemore, S. J. (2010). The developing social brain: Implications for education. *Neuron, 65*(6), 744–747. https://doi.org/10.1016/j.neuron.2010.03.004

Cahapay, M. B. (2020). How Filipino parents home educate their children with autism during COVID-19 period. *International Journal of Developmental Disabilities.* https://doi.org/10.1080/20473869.2020.1780554

Cortese, S., Asherson, P., Sonuga-Barke, E., Banaschewski, T., Brandeis, D., Buitelaar J., Coghill, D., Daley, D., Danckaerts, M., Dittmann, R. W., & Doepfner, M. (2020, June 1). ADHD management during the COVID-19 pandemic: Guidance from the European ADHD guidelines group. *The Lancet, 4*(6), 412–414. https://doi.org/10.1016/S2352-4642(20)30110-3

Mækelæ, M. J., Reggev, N., Defelipe, R. P., Dutra, N., Tamayo, R. M., Klevjer, K., & Pfuhl, G. (2021, June 10). Identifying resilience factors of distress and paranoia during the COVID-19 outbreak in five countries. *Frontiers in Psychology.* https://doi.org/10.3389/fpsyg.2021.661149

Mallik, C. I., & Radwan, R. B. (2021, February). Impact of lockdown due to COVID-19 pandemic in changes of prevalence of predictive psychiatric disorders among children and adolescents in Bangladesh. *Asian Journal of Psychiatry, 56.* https://doi.org/10.1016/j.ajp.2021.102554; www.thelancet.com/child-adolescent.

Nazirsi, A. (2020). Handle the autism spectrum condition during Coronavirus (COVID-19) stay at home period: Ten tips for helping parents and caregivers of young children. *Brain Science, 10,* 207. https://doi.org/10.3390/brainsci10040207

Nissen, J. B., Højgaard, D., & Thomsen, P.H. (2020). The immediate effect of COVID-19 pandemic on children and adolescents with obsessive compulsive disorder. *BMC Psychiatry, 20,* 511. https://doi.org/10.1186/s12888-020-02905-5

Sameck, D. R., & Hicks, B. (2014). Externalizing disorders and environmental risk: Mechanisms of gene-environment interplay and strategies for intervention. *Clinical Practice (London), 11*(5), 537–547. https://doi.org/10.2217/CPR.14.47

Tandon, M., Cardeli, E., & Luby, J. (2009, July). Internalizing disorders in early childhood: A review of depressive and anxiety disorders. *Child and Adolescent Psychiatric Clinics, 18*(3), 593–610. https://doi.org/10.1016/j.chc.2009.03.004; www.thelancet.com/child-adolescent Vol 4 June 2020, pg. 421.

Zaccari, V., D'Arienzo, M. C., Caiazzo, T., Magno, A., Amico, G., & Mancini, F. (2021). Narrative review of COVID-19 impact on obsessive-compulsive disorder in child, adolescent and adult clinical populations. *Frontiers in Psychiatry.* https://doi.org/10.3389/fpsyt.2021.673161

6 Empowering Through Solution-Focused Conversations

Context of COVID-19 Crisis

Jaseem Koorankot and Tilottama Mukherjee

The solution-focused approach

"Problem talk creates problems. Solution talk creates solutions." – The crux of the solution-focused approach lies in these words by Steve de Shazer. The solution-focused approach in therapy is an evidence-based form of psychotherapy first developed by Steve de Shazer and Insoo Kim Berg at the Brief Family Therapy Center in Milwaukee, the United States of America, in the 1980s. A plethora of researches have been conducted on how changes are brought about in the mental and physical well-being of a person in crisis in the past couple of decades. However, in the presence of more than dozens of psychotherapies, what makes the solution-focused approach stand out is its feature of filtering down the vital few from the trivial many. It is the narrowing down of the vital few questions that has the potential to bring in positive changes to the client at the earliest (Kim, Jordan, Franklin & Froerer, 2019; Macdonald, 2011).

Contrary to many other therapy models, including psychoanalytical therapies and cognitive therapies, the solution-focused approach is brief and effective and brings about instant results. Time consumption is a major differentiating factor that makes solution-focused approach advantageous over other types of therapies. To give an outline, while it is roughly 8 to 12 meetings for Cognitive Behavioural Therapy (CBT) and 40 to 80 meetings for psychoanalytical therapy, Solution-Focused Brief Therapy (SFBT) proceeds to show changes within an average of 4.5 sessions. And it was also found that there was more negative content in CBT than SFBT, and there was also a tendency for clients to respond in kind in SFBT (Jordan, Froerer & Bavelas, 2013).

What makes SFBT remarkably fast and effective is its shift from the traditional medical model approach, which emphasises recognising and treating the deeper root cause, which in turn is time consuming. Instead of digging in past traumas and finding patterns, the therapist helps the client build the

DOI: 10.4324/9781003348429-6

image of a preferred future. Moreover, this small change in perspective often encourages the client to recognise his hidden resources blurred by the magnitude of the problem. As Steve stated in the quote mentioned earlier, digging into problems creates more problems, and substituting them with a solution-focused conversation will help both the client and the therapist land at desired outcomes fast. Although the emphasis is on the future rather than the past, it is not strictly restricted to future talk. The conversations regarding the past are focused on the previous successes or, in other words, the exceptions in the conflict the client is going through. SFBT often adopts questions as interventions. They apply questions and questioning in different ways following a cognitive change (Koorankot, Rajan, Shabnam & Latheef, 2017).

The crisis

Unlike the usual stresses and conflicts that are a part of everyday life at home and work, acute crisis episodes and prolonging tough times frequently overwhelm our traditional coping skills and result in dysfunctional behaviour (Roberts, 2005). Each individual is unique, and so are their issues or, in other words, the crisis they have to tackle. A crisis comes in all forms and ways. One such global crisis we all had to face recently whose repercussions still extensively exists is the COVID-19 pandemic. The world had to come to a halt, and almost all of us got affected in one way or another. But some of us got mentally wounded massively by losing a loved one or a job or having to stay away from home. In such a situation where everyone is affected, it is not practical to give capsule-like advice or solution to the client. The therapist can only equip the client to deal with the solution better with more resources. That is where SFBT becomes ever more relevant. Among all the resources, the most non-renewable resource is, in fact, time! Once you use it, there is no going back. So, it is substantial to use it wisely and make the most out of it. SFBT has been applied to clients managing various forms of trauma (Froerer et al., 2018), focusing on post-traumatic success rather than the trauma or PTSD symptoms experienced by the client, and also it was seen that the severity of distress decreased and positive affect after SFBT (Koorankot, Mukherjee & Ashraf, 2014; Koorankot, Rajan & Ashraf, 2019).

Overview of a solution-focused meeting/therapy

Although SFBT advocates solution talks over problem talks, a problem description is vital to the session, just like any other therapy practice. However, how SFBT differs from the traditional approaches regarding the problem description is that it is entirely up to the client to decide what to share and what not to share. The therapist would not force the client to share beyond his/her capability. To be precise, digging into the problem is the differentiating factor between SFBT and other practices. Once the client describes the issue they are facing, instead of peeling more layers into the issue to decipher what and where it went wrong, the therapist helps the client set goals.

Goal formulation is the method of extracting the preferred future of the client. It helps the therapist learn what changes the client envisions for himself/herself. This preferred future is learned not by directly disposing of the question but subtly making the client picture hypothetical situations. For example the therapist can frame the question like, "So consider you are out of this trouble, how would your day look like? What all things would you succeed in doing that you fail to do now?" Instead of making the client talk about emotions and feelings and thereby creating an unrealistic future, the therapist deliberately places the question in a social context by asking about what an otherwise ordinary day would look like. According to George's (2010) article 'What about the Past?', the things we do today and tomorrow will be shaped by our preferred futures, and where we hope to end up. In that way, the client sees their life not solely by the influence of the current emotional state but from the perspective of those that surround her/him as well.

Once the destination or the goal is set, what is next is to scale the distance to that point. Scaling helps both the client and the therapist evaluate the client's current position concerning the goal set. Moreover, it pushes the client to self-evaluate, which will make them realise how much they have already progressed and that there is still room for improvement. Scaling questions can be asked like; "From a scale of 0–10, zero being you not even able to make it up to the decision to consult a therapist and 10 being your desired future outcome, where do you think you stand today?" Here, indicating that the decision to talk to a therapist is already a sign of progress boosts the client's confidence and reassures their resources. Asking questions that goes like; "How did you manage to do that?" or "What helped you to make such progress which allowed you to reach at a/ an (answered number) today?" will subtly open the door to the resources which are already with the client.

With an average of 4.5 sessions, it is ideal to have the first session where the problem description comes into play to be 40–60 minutes long and the follow-up sessions to be 20–40 minutes in length. Nevertheless, it is highly prescribed to indicate the ending of the session beforehand and not end it abruptly without warning. The ending can be subtly indicated with statements like, "Before we wind up, I have two more questions for you, is that okay with you?". In this way, the smooth flow of the conversation would not be affected by the sudden end of the session, as the client gets a hint beforehand that the session is about to end. The frequency of the follow-up sessions can then be decided according to the client. However, the therapeutic change dramatically depends upon the therapist's use of valuable questions.

The key is to make useful questions

Questions navigate the conversation. It is not an unknown fact that the conversation is the inevitable process of healing in therapy. The benefit of a good conversation is that it gives insight into a person's thought process, here, the client. Talking is one of the two best ways to get to know the thought content of a person, the other being writing. And hence the conversation is an interview in itself, and the interview itself is the intervention here. The immediate goal, apart from the long-term goal of the session thus, is to shift the negative affect of the client to a positive affect towards the end of the session. Knowing the significance of the vocabulary used is paramount in framing useful questions. For example referring to the past can be framed in one of two ways: either ask about the details of the issue while it occurred or inquire about the exceptional cases or, more precisely, the absence of the problem in recent times. By changing the focus from the problem to its absence in this instance, the therapist can light hope for change. That is to say, focus on the resources is preferred rather than any indication of the deficits. It is this key feature of the solution-focused approach that makes it more effective instantaneously. When we analyse deeper in this post-modern approach, there are three main basic principles to the solution-focused approach. In the words of de Shazer. **"If it ain't broke, do not fix it"**.

It is easy to misinterpret the given information by the client by misjudging or by quickly responding to trivial matters instead of tending to the real issue. So the recommended method is not to fix anything which does not need a fix. That is by quickly landing in conclusion regarding what the client is trying to convey.

Once you know what works, do more of it

There are three phases to a problem once it starts. The first is the phase after the problem has started. The second is the pre-morbid condition, which is the period before the issue exists. And the third is the present situation.

In a solution-focused approach, a therapist needs to, once a client comes with an issue, find what works for him by analysing the exceptions in the past and thereby finding a pattern that is a route map to the solution or, in other words, the preferred future.

The questions the therapist comes up with to learn about the client's resources before and after the onset will provide the client with awareness about one's resources.

It is very rarely that a client has a positive perspective about a crisis he/she is in. Quite often, the focus is on the issue rather than the resources or lessons they learned. So, asking the right question which turns the focus from the problem to the resources will significantly help. So, if you need to help the client, it is necessary to know what works with your client. Each client is unique, and once you know what works with them, all there is left to do is subtly suggest them to do more of it instead of giving a piece of direct advice. That is by asking questions like "How did you do that?" and "How did you manage to pull that off?" Questions like these serve two purposes; it works as a compliment and, also, it makes the client realise their resources which eventually will let them apply them in the long run.

If it does not work, do not do it again, do something different

When the client has come to you after trying or experimenting with what is supposed to be a solution, it is highly undesirable to give them the same methods to try again from a therapist's point of view. What a therapist has to do when the client says he/she has tried and failed in such and such instant solutions is help them renavigate by asking about exceptions or past successes. What is important is not to repeat what is not working.

Another approach to this is that, regardless of the successful application of the solution-focused approach, the client persists in not showing any improvement; it is best to change the therapy approach itself to any other – for example cognitive behavioural or any other approach in which the therapist is efficient. If it still does not work, it is preferred to refer the client to a different therapist.

The effectiveness of the solution-focused approach will significantly depend on the attitude of the therapist towards the client. An all-knowing attitude will adversely affect the direction as well as the result of the therapy. So, it is crucial to be the ignorant one and consider the client as the expert in his own life. Because regardless of all the technical education of the therapist, it is nearly impossible for the therapist to discern every nuance of the client's life. Instead of jumping to conclusions and building solutions over misinterpreted information and resources, be the ignorant one and have enough curiosity to listen to the client with natural empathy without being judgmental.

"The devil is always in the details"

It is easier to brush over the important stuff, but to discern the more profound meaning, the therapist will have to pay attention to each of the words and their meaning. Using the client's own words to echo and thus acknowledge the issue will reassure the client that he/she is heard and is not being judged. Once the client finishes talking about the issues, direct them to the previous successes by asking about exceptions in the recent event of the crisis.

For example

Client:	I have been having a hard time getting enough sleep since the lockdown started. I tried a lot of things to get some sleep. I stopped scrolling after 7, stopped drinking coffee, and even brought myself to bed early so that even it takes a lot of time to fall asleep, I'll get at least some sleep. But nothing seems to work. I do not know what to do!
Therapist:	Hmmm, so it is really hard for you to get some sleep these days, right? As you have mentioned, you even tried a bunch of methods, but it does not seem to work, right? (Echoing the words)
Client:	Right!
Therapist:	Since this issue started, how have you managed the situation so far? (Asking about previous success/exceptions in the issue)
Client:	Not sure, somehow managed, there were some days where I could sleep for some hours may be.
Therapist:	I see, so, what was different then? How did you do that? (Indicating the resources that's already with the client)

In this way, you are taking the focus away from the problem to the solution to which the client already has the resources. Furthermore, with the last question, you are also taking the client as the expert to their own life instead of giving readymade advice which may or may not work for them.

It is essential to provide a natural gaze and listening skills during the conversation by indicating that you are genuinely curious. However, it is not recommended to dig into every unpleasant experience which the client does not want to talk about in the name of curiosity and interest. [For example in the case of someone who has had a traumatic hospitalisation due to a COVID-19 infection and in the case of a survivor of molestation, asking about the details will push the client to relive the trauma, and that is not the recommended approach in the solution-focused approach. Instead, a neutral question should be framed, which goes like, "Is there anything that I should know as your therapist." In case of hesitation on the client's part, the therapist shall move on to the next as it is entirely up to the client to decide what to talk about. Talking about things that are not important for the client will only create more problems or push the client to relive the trauma. Another question to dig in deeper would be, "What will be the first sign when you notice things are different for you?" Besides the "what" part, "who" carries as much importance too. For instance when talking about the preferred future scenario, ask questions like, "Imagine you have lived past this crisis and have overcome all the difficulties related to this. Who do you think will notice the changes first in you?" With this, a quick study on the person/people important to the client can be done. Most of the questions aforementioned are from a not-knowing point of view. Such a perspective helps build up curiosity and opens doors for the solution quickly. On the contrary, an all-knowing attitude will end up in direct advice, which might not be the output the client desires because the path to the solution is more helpful than an instant set of advice.

The significance of asking about the "who"-question is that it places the person in a social context, making his preferred future more realistic and practical. The brain activities greatly vary when a person narrates in behavioural terms than when they narrate things standing in their feelings/emotional terms. When the person creates a mental picture of their preferred future concretely with minute details, there is a high chance that the person will end up doing that. Because that will create a prospective memory in the client's brain, and later they can pick up cues so that they will end up doing those things. When a person creates a mental picture with more clarity, that will act as a motivating factor to move towards it as well as a regulatory behaviour.

Extending SFBT towards managing the pandemic crisis

The Stockdale paradox

James Stockdale was a naval officer and Vietnam war prisoner. He has been in solitary confinement in Hanoi, Vietnam, for more than 7 years. During his time there, his fellow prisoners were quite longing to go home, and they expected to be home by the next Christmas or New Year. And every time it happened otherwise, they got more depressed and unmotivated. However, Stockdale had a different approach. He advised that it is good to be optimistic about the circumstance, but packing it with unrealistic expectations would harm our mental well-being more. For instance in the case of the pandemic, it is good to hold a hopeful dream of a world without the COVID-19 crisis, but an answer to the "when" would not be the best advice for mental well-being.

On the other hand, Stockdale insists on focusing on what is in our control and making awareness, rather than focus on what is not in our control and get worried about it. In the context of the COVID-19 crisis, staying hopeful about a COVID-19-free world and staying connected with the closed ones even when we are physically disconnected would help.

Regardless of the nature of the crisis, every crisis can be managed effectively by applying a simple statement made by Arthur Ashe, an American professional tennis player who won three Grand Slam singles titles: "Start where you are. Use what you have. Do what you can." These words have redefined the solution-focused approach. Apprehending these three subparts can result in an effective solution-focused conversation with the help seekers.

Phase 1: start where you are

The first phase of the approach can be derived from the statement, "Start where you are." Unlike the traditional approach, SFBT advocates thinking forward into the future and not backward into the past to know the root cause. Once a help seeker approaches a therapist, the therapist has to pay attention and understand what the client brings in – listening empathically to the help seeker and acknowledging and empathising with the circumstances that they are in can win the trust of the client and let them entrust you with what they want to share with you. These shared thoughts and feelings become the source of information on the help seeker's resources later. However, there are mainly three things to pay attention to when the client shares their concern.

1. Do not exaggerate the distress

Instead of adding fuel to the fire by exaggerated remarks or gestures by the therapist, acknowledge the issue with utmost care. Instead of making the "problem" bigger, receive and accept the problem as it is at its own value.

2. Do not deny the pain or suffering the client is going through

Do not try to argue people about their distress. What is important is to accept what the client brings in and not deny the pain they are going through. Denying the pain or suffering can be avoided easily by taking care of the "yes, but . . ." statement. Because "but" automatically nullifies the positive acknowledgement given just before it.

3. Do not detain the client in their distress

To bring this first phase smoothly, the therapist will have to adopt a non-expertise stance, listen for what is important for the client, and create common ground. Therapist may invite to move on in a subtle manner by not making the client to experience the pain longer than they need. One of the key skill needed in this phase as well as in the other phase of conversation is grounding skill.

Grounding

Grounding is, in short, to accept, acknowledge, and empathise with the client in every possible manner. In other words, when a speaker presents a new piece of information, the therapist accepts and indicates that he/she understood the information provided by the speaker or, here, the client. Nodding or even echoing the delivered information will let the speaker realise the addressee has got the 'idea' right"! Then it is the client's turn to acknowledge that the addressee understood it correctly. Once the speaker acknowledges it, empathise with the client by small gestures or verbal indications.

Grounding steps

1) The client presents a new information.
2) The therapist indicates or displays that he or she understood the information it (or not).
3) The client acknowledges that the addressee understood it correctly (or not).

Phase 2: use what you have

Once we move on to the next phase, the foremost important thing to do is decipher the resources that can help them through the recovery journey. To do that, the therapist will have to shift the client's focus to exceptions in the situation to identify his/her resources by retrospective resources, for example with questions like "How have you managed this situation so far?" and "Since this issue started, tell me about the time or moment where you were managing this better?" And in most cases, there will be exceptions. Once the client articulates this successful tackling that they have unknowingly done, follow it with a question that also happens to be a compliment – "How did you do that?" In this way, both the therapist and the help seeker will be able to unlock the resources with the client. The resources can either be internal or external. Which is to say, if the person in crisis had managed the issue so far by talking to a friend, that is an external resource. However, it will not be practical to indicate to do more of it in that case. So, the therapist will have to bring attention to other internal resources the client may have used. So gently point it out by asking questions like "What are the other things you decided to do, and which helped to tackle this situation?"

Similarly, questions can be framed differently to look for resources. For instance

- "Suppose that these challenging times for you have ended and you made it through! And then, you are sharing your experience with your friend with whom you have not disclosed any of this. What will you say to that friend about how you have surprised yourself with how well you coped and managed this situation?"
- "What will you say about how you made it through, and what strengths and resources you called on that were helpful to you and your family?"
- "When you survive this crisis, looking back on how you managed through, what will make you most pleased or proud about the way you did that? How do you want to be remembered?"

Creating such nuanced future questions will allow the client to see the light at the end of the tunnel, and it is highly likely that they will practice what they have said.

Phase 3: do what you can

While moving to phase three, the help provider invites the help seeker to pay attention to the expectations of beneficial change. Two types of questions are utilised here. One is preferred future question and another is scaling questions.

Preferred future questions

Preferred future questions can be framed in multiple forms. The following are some of the questions that might help to discern it.

- Suppose you woke up tomorrow, and you were somehow in your very best self despite this situation, what would you notice?

- Tomorrow or over the next few days, when you live in the best possible way despite this situation, what would you notice in yourself?
- In the coming days, what would let you know that you are doing your best in life?
- When do you hope to notice this the most? What time of the day would that be? Who else will notice this in you? What would they say about the change?
- What are your best hopes for what might be different once this tough situation has been moved?

Once the goal(s) has been set, it is vital to prioritise the goals in case there are multiple goals. Ask questions like, "Among these important set of goals that you discussed with me, what is it that you hold the most important right now?". Because it is crucial to concrete the goal to have better clarity and results.

Scaling question

We take the client forward and shift the person from an emotional state to a logical one. This shift from the emotional to the logical state is made by asking scaling questions. In this, the scaling question enables the person to think of minute steps that are required for moving ahead by using whatever the resources are available. There is a sequence for scaling question. For example:

"On a scale from 0 to 10, where '10' is a state in which you are being or making your best possible life despite of the situation, and '0' is the opposite. Where would you put yourself on the scale?"

1) What are the efforts you've already been making, that helped you to stay at – (x) in the scale?
2) How different you will be when you are at 10?
3) Who else would notice it? Or Whom do you want it to be noticed by?
4) What would they say if they noticed your changes?

"Suppose, if in coming days somehow you are making efforts to move ahead and you made a minute progress from – (x) to – (y), How different you would be when you move from 'x' to 'y'?"

1) Who else would notice it? Or Whom do you want it to be noticed by?
2) What would they say if they noticed your changes?

There are two things to pay attention to once the client answers the scaling question.

1. Compliment the person for any little progress or positive response. Ask them what made him/her say that particular number and not any lesser number. Even if the person says he/she stands on a 1, ask them what made them not say zero and how did they do that.
2. In case the help seeker persists in zero, then repeat the steps: Accept, Acknowledge, and Empathise. And take some more time doing that.

As an extension to the scaling question asks questions that hint about the preferred future. Questions like "How would it look like when you are at 10?" would help the client picture themselves in a more positive future, which will build hope and would subtly set the goal.

A small step ahead on the scale

"So, as of now, you are at a 3. What would it take you to say that you are at a 4 on the scale?" This will help the client see through the fog of their emotions and feelings and prompt them to work on it and make progress immediately. Finally, imply that the session is reaching an end so that it is not abrupt. A short statement like "I have one more question before we wind up this session!" can do that work gracefully, thus making the end of the succession smooth. And then finally, conclude the session by summarising the session and inviting their attention to the immediate activating behaviour they expect to do after the meeting and reinforcing it by natural complements. When summarising the session, get the specific points for coping questions. Organise the resources and strengths and see what the client has already achieved.

Connecting questions will help the client to connect to their behaviour. If the reaction to predicting the activating behaviour is negative or neutral, the therapist can assign homework. The concluding conversation can develop like:

Therapist: So, What act of yours will indicate that you have decided to make progress?
Client: I am not \really sure about that. I do not know!
Therapist: That is fine. I will give you homework instead. When we meet here next time, I will ask you what all have been better since our conversation. Then you may have to tell me the first thing you did to make progress and every other step as well. So you may make attempts to remember what has been better with you. Is that okay for you?

Here, we are not expecting the client to say what he/she did precisely; however, the paradoxical intention of the question is to make the client pre-plan and work on what they are going to do.

Caution: do not be solution forced, be solution-focused

When a help seeker in deep distress approaches the therapist, and he goes on talking about the problem, the best thing the therapist can do is be a good listener and empathise. Forcing a solution-focused approach on such an instance is highly undesirable and not recommended at all. That is why it is essential to be solution-focused and not solution-forced.

Summary

The first phase of the approach is derived from "Start where you are." Listening to a person seeking help to tackle his issues in these times will build a strong base for future conversations. Understanding what the person is going through and empathising with them can help them entrust you with the thoughts they want to share with you. Once the help seeker feels heard and acknowledged by the therapist or the help provider, it is time to move on to the next phase, which can be derived from "Use what you have." First, decipher what all resources which can be of use to help them through the recovery journey. Find exceptions for the person and the coping strategies the help seeker might have used in dealing with the current crisis. Frame questions that are exclusively based on them, their activities, their coping methods, and how they feel about all of it. A narration of how the help seeker handled tough times will give them a form of confidence that they lacked before.

The third phase of the conversation, derived from "Do what you can", is the most crucial part of the solution-focused conversation because this will decide what effective changes you could make in the person seeking help. Changing their emotional state to more of a logical state which is stable is the first tread in this phase. Questions regarding the minute details of the expected changes in the preferred future make the process easier and give them the clarity on how they should work on it. Next, create goals, prioritise, and break them down into more manageable steps to achieve the ultimate goal. Finally, imply that the meeting is reaching an end in order to avoid an abrupt conclusion. Conclude the session by inviting their attention to the immediate activating behaviour they expect to do after the meeting and reinforce it by natural complements. Following this three-tier method as a solution-focused approach is one of the most meaningful and effortless ways to accomplish results.

References

Bannink, F. P. (2010). *1001 solution-focused questions: Handbook for solution-focused interviewing*. Norton.

Bannink, F. P. (2015). *101 solution-focused questions for help with trauma*. Norton.

De Jong, P., & Berg, I. K. (2002). *Interviewing for solutions*. Thomson.

De Shazer, S. (1985). *Keys to solution in brief therapy*. Norton.

De Shazer, S. (1994). *Words were originally magic*. Norton.

De Shazer, S., & Dolan, Y. (2007). *More than miracles: The state of the art of solution-focused brief therapy*. The Haworth Press.

Froerer, A., von Cziffra-Bergs, J., Kim, J., & Connie, E. (Eds.). (2018). *Solution-focused brief therapy with clients managing trauma*. Oxford University Press.

George, E. (2010). What about the past? *BRIEF Forum*. www.brief.org.uk

Jordan, S. S., Froerer, A. S., & Bavelas, J. B. (2013). Microanalysis of positive and negative content in solution-focused brief therapy and cognitive behavioral therapy expert sessions. *Journal of Systemic Therapies, 32*(3), 46–59.

Kim, J., Smock Jordan, S., Franklin, C., & Froerer, A. (2019). Is solution-focused brief therapy evidence-based? An update 10 years later. *Families in Society, 100*(2), 127–138. http://dx.doi.org/10.1177/1044389419841688

Koorankot, J., Mukherjee, T., & Ashraf, Z. A. (2014). Solution-focused brief therapy for depression in an Indian tribal community: A pilot study. *International Journal of Solution-Focused Practices, 2*(1), 4–8. https://doi.org/10.14335/ijsfp.v2i1.16

Koorankot, J., Rajan, S. K., & Ashraf, Z. (2019). Solution focused versus problem focused questions: Effect on electrophysiological states and affective experiences. *Journal of Systemic Therapies, 38*, 64–78.

Koorankot, J., Rajan, S. K., Shabnam, F., & Latheef, S. A. (2017). Different types of ques- tions in psychotherapy. In *Time effective psychosocial interventions in mental health* (pp. 96–99). IMHANS.

Macdonald, A. J. (2011). *Solution-focused therapy: Theory, research & practice* (2nd ed.). Sage Publications.

Ratney, H., George, E., & Iveson, C. (2012). *Solution focused brief therapy: 100 key points and techniques*. Routledge.

Roberts, A. R. (Ed.). (2005). *Crisis intervention handbook: Assessment, treatment, and research*. Oxford University Press.

7 Concluding Remarks – Current Standing and Future Directions

Turfa Ahmed and Sukanya Chowdhury

The turn of the decade welcomed a devastating change in the guise of a global pandemic worldwide. The social distancing, quarantining, and isolation measures taken to contain the pandemic left social, psychological, economic, cultural, political, and personal ramifications in the lives of humankind. Individuals worldwide experienced several transitions in their lives because of the lockdowns imposed worldwide. Confinement in the household, working from home, financial instability, loss of jobs, closure of schools, online classes, increased burden of care on women, and a host of other distinctive problems have blurred the boundaries between an individual's personal space and their life shared with others. Issues like these have given rise to a host of Mental Health problems among individuals of all age groups, which has enhanced the value of seeking Mental Health support from professionals.

Chapter 1 discussed the trend of Mental Health literacy in India and found that stigma still exists among young adults regarding mental illness, leading to less empathy towards persons with mental illness. Age has also been significantly associated with attitude towards mental illness and emotional intelligence. *Chapter 2* discussed practicing health behaviour and health beliefs in an Indian culture-specific context of a global pandemic. The authors asserted the importance of health beliefs held by adults in influencing the susceptibility and severity of the disease perceived, the pros and cons of practicing healthy behaviours, and the individuals' self-efficacy in maintaining community health protocols during the global pandemic.

Chapter 3 highlighted the impact of the pandemic on the quality of life, general health, and resilience among an adult sample. The study highlights the differences in the indices mentioned earlier of Mental Health between individuals who contracted the SARS-CoV-2 virus and those who did not contract the disease. The results showed that those who did not contract the disease had a significantly low Mental Health index compared to the survivors of COVID-19, which was hypothesised to be due to the consistent

DOI: 10.4324/9781003348429-7

survival struggles, which might have led individuals to overlook their Mental Health difficulties. *Chapter 4* ignited a discussion about the elephant in the room: loneliness during the pandemic. The chapter explains the role of adaptive and maladaptive emotional strategies on students' psychological well-being during the pandemic. It was found that social and emotional components associated with loneliness are negatively related to psychological well-being and have been found to predict the latter significantly.

The management of children suffering from Mental Health issues during the pandemic, particularly with neurodevelopmental problems such as autism spectrum disorders and Attention Deficit Disorders (ADD), was the focus of *Chapter 5*. The chapter presented a review of studies that dealt with challenging children and suggested the management protocols for such children. Indeed, the pandemic has proven to be more difficult to deal with in families of children with special needs, with an enormous share of responsibilities on the families, particularly the parents of such children, to nurture their childhood and help them adapt to the new normal brought in by the pandemic. *Chapter 6* reported using solution-focused approaches for Mental Health interventions during the pandemic. The authors introduced the three phases of the intervention process that would help individuals start having Mental Health conversations empathically, using their repository of resources to practice solution-focused strategies in bringing about an affirmative change in their lives.

Mental Health problems and their associated behavioural disorders affect more than 10% of the adult population worldwide in any given year. For several mental disorders, the onset is during young adulthood, the most productive period of a person's life, thus leading to a prolonged diminished quality of living. Not only the patient's quality of life is affected, but it also takes a heavy toll on the family members and caregivers of the mentally ill. Families bear various social costs, such as the emotional burden of tending to family members with mental disorders, stigmatisation, and exclusion from social circles, deprived of opportunities for self-improvement in the future. Most countries do not have public-funded insurance schemes for the treatment costs for mental disorders; in such cases, families have to bear a significant amount of the economic costs, which adds to the already existing burden of social stigma and ostracisation.

However, India has been in a Mental Health crisis for a long time now, which COVID-19 is now exacerbating. Statistics for mental disorders in India show the prevalence rates ranging from 10 to 370 per 1000 population all over the country (Reddy & Chandrashekhar, 1998; Murali, 2001). Illiteracy, lack of awareness, absence of healthcare facilities, the stigma surrounding Mental Health, and delayed help-seeking behaviour are some of the causal factors for the Mental Health crisis in India. Access to adequate

Mental Health care is affected because mental illness is still not well understood and is often ignored. The mentally ill, their families and friends, and doctors and other health officials providing care are still stigmatised. These attitudes are deep-rooted in the society from which we come. Mental illness is often looked at with fear of potential threats from the patients themselves. This fear, coupled with medical ignorance, gives rise to a negative attitude, with insufficient focus on a patient's medical needs. A majority of the population perceives mental illness as incurable or self-inflicted by a patient's life choices. Beliefs can also damage a patient's chance of being referred for appropriate Mental Health treatment (Kishore, 2004). As per an article published in the *Economic Times* in 2018, in a report released by the Ministry of State for Health and Family Welfare, India has 3,827 psychiatrists against the 13,500 required and only 898 psychologists present against the 20,250 required. These figures give an insight into the absence of proper Mental Health care services.

In a country that already has a lack of resources to deal with the Mental Health crisis, COVID-19 has just made the situation grimmer since its arrival. The pandemic and subsequent lockdowns have led to many complaints about Mental Health. The common Mental Health issues that have been reported to be related to the current pandemic globally are anxiety, insomnia, denial, frustration, fatigue, anger, fear, and melancholy (Torales et al., 2020). An article published in *JAMA Psychiatry* reports that COVID-19 may increase the risk of suicide (Xiang et al., 2020). There have been reports of COVID-19-related suicide-related death in India in Maharashtra, Uttar Pradesh, Assam, and Kerala (Cullen et al., 2020). A few prominent celebrity suicides have been reported during this period as well. According to an article published in *The Wire* in December 2020, there was a 67% increase in suicidal behaviour during the pandemic, post the nationwide lockdown. There have been consistent reports of the suicide of healthcare workers, migrant labourers, and patients in quarantine centres since the pandemic. In a study conducted on the frontline medical health professionals in the country, doctors and nurses reported feeling depressed, experiencing sleep disturbances, increased irritability and restlessness, and a fear of contracting COVID-19. Seventeen per cent of the respondents reported feeling the need for a psychological consultation for themselves, 3.4% wanted a consultation for members of their families, whereas another 3.4% wanted a consultation for both themselves and the members of their family (Roy et al., 2021).

The UNICEF and the Gallup organisation conducted a survey in the early months of 2021 among 20,000 children and adults in 21 countries, and the survey findings are previewed in *The State of the World's Children 2021*. Among them, only 41 per cent of the population in India, ranging from 15 to

24 years of age, said that it is good to seek treatment for Mental Health problems, compared to an average of 83 per cent who felt the same from the 21 countries. India also was the only country where a minority of young adults felt that people suffering from Mental Health problems should seek help. Other countries had most young adults (56–95 per cent) feeling that reaching out for help was a big step in dealing with Mental Health problems. The study also found that around 14% of 15- to 24-year-olds in India reported feeling often depressed or having little-to-no interest in carrying out their day-to-day activities.

While the world is dealing with one pandemic, we have another hidden pandemic with severe, long-lasting effects that will cripple society for years to come. A lack of experiential knowledge of dealing with mental disorders, lack of proper healthcare facilities, lack of staff, lack of compliance on the part of the patients and their families, and general apathy of the society towards the mentally ill have over the years, giving rise to this pandemic. Countering its effects needs collective effort by various stakeholders located at different levels of society, including government officials, community health workers, people dealing with mental illness, their families, police, non-governmental organisations, and policymakers. A sincere effort needs to be channelled towards developing new infrastructure related to Mental Health care needs, which can deal with the crisis at the institutional and community levels and aim to expand the existing available resources continuously.

A study (Ahuja et al., 2020) affirmed that the pandemic had given birth to fear, anxiousness, despair, stress, and other kinds of psychological distress among most individuals around the globe. The fear of contracting the virus and subsequent life-threatening suffering have left no alternative for the communities but to fight back by ensuring social distancing and quarantine procedures whenever required and facilitating recovery for those who have contracted the disease. Social support from agents such as spouses or other family members plays an indispensable role during public health emergencies by decreasing the mental weight and providing social help and help-seeking techniques, thereby proving resilience in adversity. Thus, social support has been reported to have a negative association with perceived stress during the pandemic and served more as a predictor of stress than a protector from stress (Uddin et al., 2022). A recent study also found that engaging in social distancing behaviours gives an opportunity to develop resilience among individuals (Panzeri et al., 2021), and long-term exposure to multiple adverse stressors such as the shroud of the uncertainty of the pandemic over various domains of life such as career plans, personal and occupational lives, and looming apprehension of the spread of infection at the community level not only might have been daunting but also offered a chance to nurture one's resilience (known as the *steeling effect*; Seery et al., 2010).

Humans are social beings, and the sense of connectedness that individuals share amongthemselves comes forth through the physical environment. With the advent of the imposition of nationwide lockdown, individuals had no choice but to become restricted in the confines of their domestic life. Work and life balance became highly blurred, and proximity with just the family members was a source of tension within the household and mental space. The source of respite that the individuals had in their social areas outside their homes was lost overnight. This aggravated feelings of loneliness, helplessness, and apprehensions concerning their upcoming professional, educational, or personal lives. This has also been corroborated by a recent preliminary study conducted by researchers at Harvard University (Weissbourd et al., 2021), which confirms that loneliness is at elevated levels, especially among young adults due to the pandemic. Whether the loneliness is experienced due to the longing for support and connections with loved ones in a pre-pandemic world, not having enough friends to share one's state of mind, losing their loved ones to the fatalities of the COVID-19 virus, or feeling unheard or unacknowledged by others – loneliness can stem from numerous sources. The study also highlighted the importance of the people, who felt that they are "genuinely cared for" by others – demonstrated by their approach to the overtures of the individual. If that is not met adequately, it starts a vicious loop where the individual tends to feel rejected and self-critical for expecting to receive that concern from others, which aggravates the shame one has around the notion of suffering from Mental Health concerns and thereby leading them to withdraw from seeking any social support and, thus, lowering the mental well-being of the individual. All such factors are intricately woven into the determination of the quality of life of an individual.

Social media further aggravates the feelings of dejection and isolation because of the deluge of posts from people, which falsely portray versions of grandiose lifestyles and exaggerated presence of social support in some cases, which exacerbates the individuals' worsening Mental Health (Weissbourd et al., 2021). Thus, the likelihood of developing emotional loneliness among individuals over time stems from their social loneliness. Lonely individuals tend to have fewer individuals in their lives with whom they share their private matters or turn for help. These factors played a crucial role during the pandemic (Lampraki et al., 2022). In the Indian context, a review of studies had a parallel account to narrate (Banerjee & Rai, 2020) that loneliness is one of the primary factors that lead to social isolation and the development of anxiety, depression, stress-related concerns, or other physical co-morbidities. The disconnection in the social lives of individuals with the advent of the global pandemic could be considered one of the primary factors that initiated a sense of loss of purpose and boredom due to the distancing measures during the lockdown period. A recent study (Fukase et al., 2021) reported that persons with depression use ineffective coping strategies such as behavioural disconnection and blaming oneself instead of effective coping strategies such as the use of problem-focussed strategies such as seeking instrumental support and planning, and denial. Denial was found to be effective only in situations where the stressor was prolonged, even though it is listed as a dysfunctional coping mechanism because it assists the individual in dealing with the stressor. Thus, persons suffering from pandemic-related psychological distress are more often than not inclined to use ineffective coping strategies.

The homebound situation of the individuals also opened the window of opportunity for some individuals to pursue creative endeavours such as art or music that would stimulate their mind and self-expression and foster social connections during the pandemic. Participation in leisure, physical, and creative activities thus is a contributor to well-being during the pandemic (Morse et al., 2021).

The pandemic has been equally distressing for children and adolescents with special needs. They have uncertainty intolerance, and the changing environment due to the imposition of restrictions exacerbates their symptoms as there is an incongruency between their current and previous routines. Dissatisfaction with the online medium of instruction was prominently reported by one of the recent studies (Maftei et al., 2022) because of the poor scope of interaction online. Thus, the pandemic was perceived to have adverse effects on children and adolescents. Even though they had learnt social-adaptive skills, there are possibilities of relapse to their past behaviours because of the lack of access to peers, resources, and opportunities for social interactions that could further their learning of behavioural and social skills which their schools or day care centres were able to provide. Their symptoms may manifest as struggles to follow instructions, comprehend the pandemic's gravity, and perform their daily chores independently (Lee, 2020). Such situations can also aggravate temper tantrums and outbursts and lead to conflict between them and their parents. The limited expertise of the parents in handling difficult children and adolescents on their own makes it even more challenging for them, who earlier used to be managed and assisted by trained professionals from schools or other institutes of concern (Dalton et al., 2020).

To survive a pandemic and heal from its post-traumatic effects, it is not enough to only highlight the severe impact it has left behind but to equally focus on the management strategies that will help us cope with the long-lasting effects it will have for years to come. Several management techniques and coping strategies to help them deal successfully with the crisis at hand. In a study, Giordano et al. (2020) examined the effectiveness of music therapy for hospital staff working in a COVID-19 virus unit at a hospital in Italy. Participants were quarantined in a hotel during the study and listened to playlists focused on energy, breathing, and serenity. The playlists were customised for each, based on their listening experience from the week before. They recorded their levels of sadness, fear, worry, and tiredness before and after listening to the playlists made for them. The study reported improvements in the four symptoms, especially in the case of the energy playlist. Music is an effective tool that helps people deal with stressful life situations. Playing a musical instrument, attending virtual music concerts, or just listening to music while doing daily chores are how people have coped with these distressing times, as highlighted by one of the chapters in this book. Music is available on a wide scale at low costs and is enjoyed by many people (Schäfer et al., 2013). Using these benefits can prove quite advantageous, especially for vulnerable groups.

Past pandemics such as Ebola have shown the efficacy of psychoeducation and Cognitive Behaviour Therapy to decrease anxiety, depression, and PTSD and improve sleep patterns, resulting in well-being and improving the quality of relationships (Waterman et al., 2018). If carried out under the guidance of a licensed Mental Health professional, such intervention techniques can help bring some betterment to the lives of those whose Mental Health has been severely affected in the past months.

A study conducted in Guandong, China, revealed the impact of individual consultation on inpatients with suspected COVID-19 who were in quarantine wards of a hospital, China (Zhou et al., 2020). The intervention involved 10-minute consultations twice a day with an onsite nurse who provided information about the situation and virtual support. Towards the end of the intervention, there were significant improvements in their anxiety and depressive symptoms (Zhou et al., 2020). These studies reveal that talking to Mental Health professionals, even for a small amount of time, changes our cognitive abilities and attitude. Social isolation, separation from loved ones, halting of educational institutions, adopting repeated preventive measures, financial troubles, unemployment have been identified as significant stressors during this pandemic. Seeking professional guidance can help us to deal with these more effectively.

Proper attention should be given to the needs of vulnerable groups such as the elderly, children, immuno-compromised individuals, survivors of abuse, incarcerated persons, institutionalised, and people with pre-existing mental illnesses. It would be more difficult for them to survive in a post-COVID-19 world. Hence, special care for such individuals should be taken.

The Government of India has taken some effective measures to tackle the Mental Health crisis in the country during COVID-19. The National Institute of Mental Health and Neurosciences (NIMHANS) worked closely with the Ministry of Health and Family Welfare setting up a task force in Mental Health on behalf of the Ministry to deal with the situation, along with a helpline that helped in establishing a continuum of care service for patients with psychiatric problems. Teleconsultation with patients was also started, where professionals provided telemedicine and tele-counselling facilities. NIMHANS also organised a digital academy, where thousands of counsellors, nurses, and other professionals are trained to provide psychosocial support in this crisis.

To overcome the life-altering effects of this pandemic, it should be ensured that Mental Health services are integrated into the COVID-19 health care response plan. This will provide adequate treatment and care for those who are psychologically disturbed due to this pandemic. Policy formulation keeping in mind effective strategies that would easily be available to the general population is the need of the hour. The following areas should be looked into.

Provisions for telepsychiatry services should be made at every Mental Health institute providing services for individuals with mental illnesses.

- Online training programmes in telecounselling for Mental Health professionals all over the country should be organised – a code of conduct, ethics, and rules should be laid down by professional bodies that can serve as the guiding principle for all Mental Health professionals.
- The Mental Health professional associations and government bodies should assemble experts with knowledge and training in psychological first aid and the management of post-traumatic psychological crises.
- Emergency interventions and management strategies for the psychological crisis should be integrated into the broad framework of pandemic prevention and control to reduce potential psychological damage arising from the pandemic and subsequent lockdown and quarantine processes.
- Policies involving special intervention techniques for the high-risk and marginalised population should be put into place to guarantee more excellent social stability.
- Primary Mental Health education as a part of the school and college curriculum for the general population must be planned to help in removing the stigma associated with mental disorders in general.

An empathetic understanding of the Mental Health and social status of different groups, especially marginalised sections of the society and how they are affected by this pandemic, is the need of the hour. Having more conversations about Mental Health at our homes, among social circles, and in workplaces is essential to breaking the taboo. Timely identifying symptoms among those around us, especially those with prior Mental Health issues, can help prevent suicides and life-threatening impulsive behaviour. The physical effects of this pandemic might start to wear off in a few years, but its long-term Mental Health effects will last for years to come, leading to severe post-traumatic symptoms and inter-generational trauma. The only way the human race can move forward from this is to pay as much attention to healing our minds as we do for our bodies.

References

Ahuja, K., Srivastava, P., & Gul, A. (2020). Resilience, well being and marital adjustment: A comparative study between those who are working from home to the ones who are working from their workplace. *Indian Journal of Mental Health*, *7*(4), 338–342.

Banerjee, D., & Rai, M. (2020). Social isolation in COVID-19: The impact of loneliness. *International Journal of Social Psychiatry*, *66*, 525–527.

Cullen, W., Gulati, G., & Kelly, B. D. (2020). Mental health in the COVID-19 pandemic. *QJM: Monthly Journal of the Association of Physicians*, *113*(5), 311–312.

Dalton, L., Rapa, E., & Stein, A. (2020). Protecting the psychological health of children through effective communication about COVID-19. *The Lancet: Child & Adolescent Health*, *4*(5), 346–347.

Fukase, Y., Ichikura, K., Murase, H., & Tagaya, H. (2021). Depression, risk factors, and coping strategies in the context of social dislocations resulting from the second wave of COVID-19 in Japan. *BMC Psychiatry*, *21*, 33.

Giordano, F., Scarlata, E., & Baroni, M. (2020). Receptive music therapy to reduce stress and improve wellbeing in Italian clinical staff involved in COVID-19 pandemic: A preliminary study. *Art Psychotherapy*, *70*, 1–5.

Kishore, J. (2004). Schizophrenia: Myths and reality. *Rationalist Voice*, 23–26.

Lampraki, C., Hoffman, A., Roquet, A., & Jopp, D. S. (2022). Loneliness during COVID-19: Development and influencing factors. *PLoS One*, *17*(3), e0265900.

Lee, J. (2020). Mental health effects of school closures during COVID-19. *The Lancet: Child & Adolescent Health*, *4*(6), 421.

Maftei, A., Merlici, I. A., & Roca, I. C. (2022). Implications of the COVID-19 pandemic on children and adolescents: Cognitive and emotional representations. *Children*, *9*, 359. www.mohfw.gov.in/pdf/COVID19Final2020ForOnline-9July2020.pdf

Morse, K. F., Fine, P. A., & Friedlander, K. J. (2021). Creativity and leisure during COVID-19: Examining the relationship between leisure activities, motivations, and psychological well-being. *Frontiers in Psychology*, *12*, 609967.

Murali, M. S. (2001). Epidemiological study of prevalence of mental disorders in India. *Indian Journal of Community Medicine*, *9*, 34–38.

Panzeri, A., Bertamini, M., Butter, S., Levita, L., Gibson-Miller, J., Vidotto, G., Bentall, R. P. & Bennett, K. M. (2021). Factors impacting resilience as a result of exposure to COVID-19: The ecological resilience model. *PLoS One, 16*(8), e0256041.

Reddy, M. V., & Chandrashekhar, C. R. (1998). Prevalence of mental and behavioural disorders in India: A meta-analysis. *Indian Journal of Psychiatry, 40,* 149–157.

Roy, A., Singh, A. K., Mishra, S., Chinnadurai, A., Mitra, A., & Bakshi, O. (2021). Mental health implications of COVID-19 pandemic and its response in India. *The International Journal of Social Psychiatry, 67*(5), 587–600.

Schäfer, T., Sedlmeier, P., Städtler, C., & Huron, D. (2013). The psychological functions of music listening. *Frontiers in Psychology, 4*(511), 1–33.

Seery, M. D., Holman, E. A., & Silver, R. C. (2010). Whatever does not kill us: Cumulative lifetime adversity, vulnerability, and resilience. *Journal of Personality and Social Psychology, 99*(6), 1025–1041.

Torales, J., O'Higgins, M., Castaldelli-Maia, J. M., & Ventriglio, A. (2020). The outbreak of COVID-19 coronavirus and its impact on global mental health. *International Journal of Social Psychiatry,* 3–6.

Uddin, M. K., Islam, M. N., & Ahmed, O. (2022). COVID-19 concern and stress in Bangladesh: perceived social support as a predictor or protector. *Trends in Psychology,* 1–17. www.unicef.org/india/press-releases/unicef-report-spotlights-mental-health-impact-covid-19-children-and-young-people

Waterman, S., Hunter, E. C. M., Cole, C. L., Evans, L. J., Greenberg, G. J., & Beck, A. (2018). Training peers to treat Ebola centre workers with anxiety and depression in Sierra Leone. *International Journal of Social Psychiatry, 64,* 156–165.

Weissbourd, R., Batanova, M., Lovison, V., & Torres, E. (2021). *Loneliness in America how the pandemic has deepened an epidemic of loneliness and what we can do about it.* Making Caring Common Project. https://static1.squarespace.com/static/5b7c56e255b02c683659fe43/t/6021776bdd04957c4 557c212/1612805995893/Loneliness+in+America+2021_02_08_FINAL.pdf https://thewire.in/health/suicides-covid-19-lockdown

Xiang, Y. T., Jin, Y., & Cheung, T. (2020). Joint international collaboration to combat mental health challenges during the coronavirus disease 2019 pandemic. *JAMA Psychiatry,* 1–2.

Zhou, L., Xie, R., Yang, X., Zhang, S., Li, D., & Zhang, Y. (2020). Feasibility and preliminary results of effectiveness of social media-based intervention on the psychological wellbeing of suspected COVID-19 cases during quarantine. *The Canadian Journal of Psychiatry,* 1–3.

Index

Page numbers in *italics* indicate a figure and page numbers in **bold** indicate a table on the corresponding page.

9781032225616